To Helen,
Hope you enjoy
Blessings

The Druid
in the Greenhouse

First published 2023

Copyright © Des Lamb 2023

The right of Des Lamb to be identified as the author of this work has been asserted in accordance with the Copyright, Designs & Patents Act 1988.

All rights reserved. No part of this book may be reproduced, stored in a retrieval system, or transmitted in any form or by any means, digital, electronic, electrostatic, magnetic tape, mechanical, photocopying, recording or otherwise, without the written permission of the copyright holder.

Published under licence by Brown Dog Books and
The Self-Publishing Partnership Ltd, 10b Greenway Farm, Bath Rd,
Wick, nr. Bath BS30 5RL, UK

www.selfpublishingpartnership.co.uk

ISBN printed book: 978-1-83952-730-2
ISBN e-book: 978-1-83952-731-9

Cover design by Andrew Prescott
Internal design by Andrew Easton

Printed and bound in the UK

This book is printed on FSC® certified paper

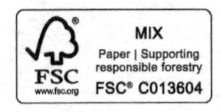

The Druid
in the Greenhouse

Des Lamb

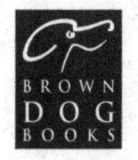

BROWN DOG BOOKS

CONTENTS

Foreword		7
1.	The House of Learning	9
2.	Gypsies, Skylarks & the Pull to the East	24
3.	Satanic Mills and the Mahatma	40
4.	Sunny Day	46
5.	Free-Falling and the Wicker Man	51
6.	Pop Music and the Turning to the East	62
7.	Universal Life Force	71
8.	Sands of Time and the Widening Approach	75
9.	Flat Top, the Facing Up and the Coming Out	87
10.	Wireline Man	92
11.	Pies for Lunch and the Weather Was Good	100
12.	Quiet before the Desert Storm	103
13.	One Starry Night Out	116
14.	The Sushumna Experience	120
15.	The Little Book of Awakening	135
16.	Poltergeist in the Staff House and the Queen's Lodge	150
17.	Barefooting on Sands of New Beginnings	163
18.	Bridges and Funeral Pyres	199
19.	Albion Return	213

20	Deep Words and Yew School Teachers	216
21	Self-Cherishing and Overcoming Obstacles	228
22	Circles in the Spirit Realm	242
23	Shades of Green Lightness	270
24	The Secret Valley	279
25	The Final Phase is Only the Beginning	286
26	The Knowing of the Known	299

FOREWORD

It was the second week of the new millennium. The place a bungalow in southern Kerala, and whilst taking daily siesta, I laid down my intention to write a book.

We may often hear it said 'If only I knew then what I know now' would we make the same mistakes again? Well maybe, as a lot would still depend upon impulse and our present thoughts and actions.

I consider myself fortunate to be born at a time of new beginnings, the period following two world wars, the opening of doors to a cultural revolution, one we simply call the sixties.

As expected, there were a few hiccups along the way, but generally things were pretty good. However, in present times the pencil appears to have sharpened. A more serious approach, although by now with further knowledge and understanding we should have created a more laid-back lifestyle, one in tune, as we sit peacefully beneath the tree of harmony.

My objective for writing this book is to tell my story, a path seeking personal growth, an awakening to some, a sharing with others on similar paths, but within its contents, adventure within the worlds, those places of darkness, amongst that of light.

Mine is not to preach or even teach, but hopefully to make one think, an opening to a realisation, as we climb the ladder of spiritual attainment.

It started as a young boy at play, some may say, living and acting out his creative thoughts on a stage of his own making.

And as the wizard child stepped out into the mighty forests of learning, crossing that great ocean of experience, he survived, and on arriving at the gates of his destiny, hung a welcome sign for you to enter

THE HOUSE OF LEARNING

Early one morning, within the cycle of the sun, the twins were in play, and within earshot of the sounds of an awakening tram shed, I arrived in the breech position, a route of entry not uncommon in those days.

Born at a time when the reign of George VI was nearing completion, and with the nation still in the recovery position from the perils of war. Wrapped in a bundle of swaddling clothes, I was taken to live with my parents and in-laws. In common with children the world over, I spent the first six months in a state of non-awareness, simply digesting, nappy filling and sleeping. And as the wheel of the year slowly turned into wintertime, like a cat on a garage roof, I began to observe the actions of others.

Those strange shapes that moved around until a recognisable face grew familiar, changes from light into darkness, the use of hands, those first realisations of likes and dislikes. Carried around, grabbing at table lamps, newspapers, and pens, and when placed on the floor, in tortoise mode set off under table and chairs, mindlessly picking and placing discarded objects into the mouth.

Layers of thick white cotton created bowed legs that made the wobbly dash across the room even more difficult, whilst constantly having to react to the name of NO can be so frustrating.

But in time and in tune with the ancients, having taken to the upright position, as the artist starts with blank canvas, so too the process of creating my very own personality, that unique sense of me, a character began to form. Yet it would take many a worn-out shoe before I developed an understanding of that one.

We lived in a fairly large house within a market garden area; at the rear of the property rows of sand-grown lettuce waved and danced to the motion of the breeze. And with a couple of glasshouses providing a home for commercially grown tomatoes, it created a dinner-table setting for many a small creature, like those of the slithering kind, the furry-legged ones, and the visiting winged variety. The rear of the plot had a border with a tree-lined dyke, and with horses living in the fields beyond, provided the setting for playful adventure.

My mother's grandad and her aunt ran a small fruit and vegetable business, and whilst my father worked for a nationalised industry, Mum stayed at home to look after me. She had a strange title of 'housewife' bestowed upon her.

It was a time of new beginnings, and one day I recall getting the full treatment. At first, I was dunked into deep bath water, and once wiped down, had a dreadful green solution combed into my longish blond hair. I was slipped into a suit with an ER logo, and on gazing into a full-length mirror, it reflected a vision of a young dude in a magazine for softies. And if that wasn't bad enough, I was whisked away to a busier location, ushered into a room, where I was instructed to stand before a man with a large white umbrella and a box on legs. As a group looked on, I was subjected to a round of flashing lights. All this because a lady that rode a horse in London was having a crown placed upon her head. And in common with many, for the decades that followed, the photograph sat in a large gold-coloured frame, a place of honour on Mum's front room cabinet, a something that mothers do. I also recall the mums getting excited when news broke that war time restrictions had eased, and bent yellow tubes called bananas arrived in the shops.

And that only caused more pain, for one day whilst standing at a bus stop for the return journey home from town, a packed bus arrived and we were informed by the conductor that there were only a few seats left vacant on the top deck. For me that was exciting, but not so for Mum. On receiving her instructions, I climbed the stairs, and on reaching the summit, entered into an adult world, one full of sights, noise, and cigarette smoke.

It was all a new experience, and as the bellowing voice of the conductor instructed us to move down the bus, we managed to find one empty aisle seat. Throughout the journey I was fascinated by the actions of the adults, I did hear a whisper that they had been drinking, a phrase new to me, but although they were very loud, they seemed rather funny. Upon further gazing around the top deck, like a draw-tube telescope my senses tuned in, for right there only a few seats directly in front lay a lovely bowl of fruit. There were apples and pears and even a grape or two, but it was the bright yellow banana that caught my eye. On scanning the horizon, the adults were either giggling or busy talking, and with a rising desire that would not go away, I became completely focused on the yellow shape. By now I had already developed the initial stages of being canny, for I knew I would have to wait for the right moment, and that came with a loud shout from the burly conductor. As Mum rose, she carried me down the aisle towards the stairs, and as I dangled below her right arm, like a tiger stalking its prey in long grass, I struck my target with force, gripping the banana as hard as I could.

With the motion of Mum moving through the bus came an almighty scream, I was determined to keep hold. Then suddenly, like the arrival of Jack from his box, the whole fruit bowl came towards me, and below, the sight of a crimped face, one with a look of anger that continued to shout, 'It's pinned!' It was anarchy on the number 6 bus, people jumped up in the aisles, the lady that lived below the fruit bowl was down on her knees.

At this point my mother was shouting. The bus stopped. The conductor came running up the stairs, and as he grabbed hold of the lady's arm, I reluctantly loosened my grip. It all ended with an incredibly angry red-faced fruit lady, climbing up from the floor, and a very embarrassed mother, whilst everyone else had gone into fits of laughter. On arrival at the bottom of the stairs, the smiling conductor told my apologetic mum, 'Don't worry, love. What do you expect a child to do if the lady is foolish enough to go out wearing a hat, which mimics a bowl of fruit.'

THE DRUID IN THE GREENHOUSE

Interestingly I recently went to one of those bygone places, where I saw a fruit bowl hat displayed on a stand; however, the banana looked a bit waxy. I resisted the temptation to grab, but it sure made me smile.

Further relaxations of post-war restrictions and the advancement of technology signalled the start of a new era, as small black and white televisions became a feature in British households.

Apart from constantly asking questions 'why and how' everything around me seemed to work, and I was aware of change. In the evenings, the adults of the house had begun to sit huddled together around the 'box' and in order to attract the children, the afternoons featured a programme called *Watch with Mother*.

At a specified time, each day, I was reluctantly ushered into position.

That first fix, a daily exposure to puppetry with a likeable mule called Muffin, followed by a communal act with a pyjama-clad boy called Andy, who lived in a basket with his pig-tailed girlfriend and a friendly cuddly bear.

I too became hooked.

Comics and children's annuals were popular, my favourite being the adventures of Rupert, a colourful bear, who lived in a magical village called Nutwood.

Rupert had lots of chums including a badger, an old goat, a Gypsy boy, and a woodland troll named Raggety. Adventures were had when they set off to meet a Chinese girl called Tiger Lily, her father the Conjurer and a dragon friend named

Ming. Together they travelled on quests to faraway lands with mystical names, like the Kingdom of Birds, and King Frost's Castle. With the stories of Rupert told at bedtime, it was the further adventures into the dream world, which enhanced my awakening. Being an only child with a vivid imagination, I had plenty of time and space to be creative. With a sprinkling of the herb of naughtiness tossed into the talking bowl, the spoon of learning began to work its magic. With an early life fascination for sticks, I had discovered a special staff; it was around my height in length and had the power to do many things. I carried it everywhere, to the dinner table, to the bathroom and even to bed, and I got frustrated when informed that for some strange reason I could not take it on a bus. But being difficult to conceal, I had to concede on that one.

In the time that followed, I heard tell of a master magician, who came from the lands across the eastern mountain range, the one that the adults called the Pennines. He appeared on our tiny screens, surprisingly another bear, who answered to the dark name of Sooty.

Sooty was a conjurer, who had a magic wand, and on uttering sacred words could make things disappear and reappear. Many a fortunate child, including myself, had a handheld version, which came in a box complete with a wand of magic, and so it began. For it was during the months of summertime I ventured out into the rear of the garden and having discovered how to open the door to the larger glasshouse, I was taken aback by a surging wave of damp pungent heat. With staff in hand, I made my way into the unknown territory, and with a slight feeling of fear, I passed unnoticed through the avenues of ripening tomatoes. With a quick scan around I noticed that tucked away in the back corner were a couple of potting benches, and on the ground below lay a pile of pots of various sizes. Beside them was an open box containing a collection of garden tools, including scissors and string.

With rising confidence, it became a daily ritual to visit the house of glass, and once inside I proceeded to place cut-out images of my friends upon the wooden bench. With Sooty's wand in hand, I learnt how to direct new adventures for Rupert and his magical friends, Tiger Lily, the trolls and the dragon, and with creative thought and intention, the practice evolved with each secret session, as more ingredients were added into the simmering brew.

New characters arrived on the TV screen in the form of Bill and Ben the Flowerpot Men, a pair that stroked the rim of the esoteric singing bowl of early learning. They were likeable lads, who lived inside two terracotta pots at the rear of a potting shed, and they had a friendly ally named Weed.

Weed the watcher, whom I assumed was a girl, lived in the space between their pots, and on signalling all clear, the pair climbed out, and whilst Weed listened and scanned the garden, many a mischievous adventure was there to be had.

When the man who lived in the big house stepped out, Weed would shout a warning that he was on his way to the garden. With a quick scramble, the men of pot would rush back, and with seconds to spare entered their homes of residence once more. Amazingly Bill and Ben grew up to become national icons. Today both can be found on display in numerous garden centres, and with many a private garden providing a home for the magical pair, the power of their spirit lives on. Having become inspired, and with the benefit of living in similar surroundings, and with the ease to travel like the bears of magic, with staff in hand I continued my adventures to the faraway land inside the Kingdom of Glass.

During the summer holidays I lived in a timeless world, for during the day I was only called in to the house to wash, eat, and on occasions got dragged to the shops. On an auspicious day of entry, I selected two large plant pots, one for Bill and one for Ben, and a medium-sized pot for Weed.

I then set about creating the potted pair from pieces of wood, cane sticks and bits of cloth. Their faces were yellow flowers taken from the rear garden, whilst Weed came from a plot at the side of the driveway. On cutting to shape and tying with string, they appeared and felt almost lifelike.

A while later whilst outside on manoeuvres, I discovered that the man from the house had left behind a number of dirt-covered glass panels, and on closer inspection some were good, whilst others were cracked with corners missing. On selecting the best, I carried them inside, using the contents of a watering can too wash them down, before wiping one side clean with my shirt sleeve, no doubt. And like a set from *Gulliver's Travels*, I placed them around the sides of the potting table, thus creating a mirror-like effect. Being a cloudless day the hot bright light from the sun cascaded down through the upper panes of the glass roof, illuminating the stage with its dazzling, shimmering golden light. Once everyone was in place, I went about dressing myself in special clothing, ceremonial garments created from a discarded grandad shirt and old sacks. And with Sooty's wand in hand, energy doth flow, words of magic spoken, and with three taps, they all came to life; of course, we all promised to keep it a secret. Then one day whilst fully immersed in a journey into the enchanted realm of trolls and dragons, I was suddenly disturbed, jerked back into reality by the sound of a loud scream, and a crash. As I turned round, through the haze, I caught sight of my aunt, standing startled and shaken in the doorway of the greenhouse. She said she was sorry, as she thought that I was something else. Then without further words she turned and scuttled away sharply back to the house, leaving a tray and a broken bowl on the ground.

I immediately brought the session to a halt and quickly followed her to the kitchen. She said she knew I was just playing, but still in shock, kept repeating that she thought I was something else, although she never did explain what that something else was.

In conclusion, my aunt said she knew that I was only playing, and that opened up another view to the fundamentals of play.

As a child I had used my creative imagination to procure a magical aspect, that of bringing toys to life, and then to travel with them to an enchanted realm.

It was a few years later when I heard that my aunt was a spiritualist, and further decades passed before I learnt in personal practice what being a spiritualist meant. But on knowing that I had upset Auntie, I ceased the practice in the house of glass, and her timely intervention was the powers of the universe simply reining me in.

But not too far away from the greenhouse, I had another secret place, a sacred one beyond the dyke, within the realm of the birds. Access to the grove was limited, as the only route of passage came by a swinging rope, one secured long ago by giants, aided by a branch of a large tree. It was a haven, where the adults could only shout across, and would never dare venture.

For it was home to grasshoppers, butterflies and working bees, and as birds sang the songs of communication, prowling feral cats patrolled the undergrowth in search of mice and shrews. On occasions a group of horses came over to find some shade in the long grass beneath the trees; it was a place where I learnt to feel at home, and at one with their presence. I had names for most of them including the cats and the big tree, for whilst sitting with my back against its trunk we entered into conversation. Apart from showing symptoms of an early stage of tree-hugging, I also took to the practice of standing on my head, whether against the tree, rear of house or the bedroom wall. I had no idea where the desire came from, and neither did my mother, who at times became alarmed by my strange practices.

In association with trees, I discovered the effects of music, and my first-ever record, 'The Woody Woodpeckers Song', a 10-inch 78-rpm disc by the American artist Kay Kyser. Woody arrived in the household amongst an old suitcase full of second-hand vinyl, along with a wind-up gramophone player and a little tin box containing hundreds of small needles. And with the aid of a turning handle, I became immersed in the actions of the little bird. Woody totally captured my imagination; I observed him flying excitedly through the woodland, alerting all in the forest with the echoing sound of his being.

I loved him, he just made me feel whole, even changing Woody's needle became a pleasurable chore. That was until the day disaster struck, and like an overzealous amateur on the Isle of Man TT course, I lost concentration and allowed the disc to slip out of my hand. Free-falling, and in slow motion, it glided out of reach, and on landing edge down on the floor, cracked like an egg. I was shocked, in fact heartbroken; my friend Woody had just died, and it was all my fault, and as I burst into tears all in the green forest became still.

I guess my parents had become concerned about me playing on my own all the time, and in order to strike a balance they arranged for two children to be delivered. The day before their arrival I had noticed that some soft soil with straw wrapped in small pieces had been dumped in a large pile at the rear of the brick shed.

It was around mid-morning when a car pulled up across the driveway gates, and after initial observations, I was introduced to a boy of similar age, who like me wore the customary jumper, shirt, and short trousers, whilst his younger sister stood smiling in a flowered dress, short white socks, and leather sandals. Having shown them around, we spent some time playing inside an old car that had been left inside the back of the garage. Once the novelty had worn off, we climbed the wooden staircase to a dusty first floor. Apart from stored lengths of timber, and cobwebs in every corner, it was home to some rather large spiders. And with that in mind I went about showing my new friends a trick. Looking around the floor, I found a small stick, and on passing it to the girl, we all crouched around a large web. And with guidance from myself, she rattled the silky fabric; her action caused an immediate effect, as a huge spider came running down to investigate, and in doing, sent the now screaming girl flying down the stairs at full speed. My mother came running out, and after a calming-down process, which included a cold drink and a biscuit, it was smiles and laughter all round. Once revitalised, I proceeded to drag a set of old timber ladders from the back of the garage and placing them against the front wall of the shed, encouraged my new friends to follow me up onto the flat roof.

Standing high we paraded around like guards on a castle battlement, and once that had worn off, it became time to make our descent. With a running jump I flew off the roof, landing safely into the centre of the newly delivered soft soil, and with a little persuasion my new friends duly followed.

Even more fun was to be had when we changed the game to see who could jump the furthest, to sink the deepest, but it came to an abrupt ending, when another loud scream rang out. Only this time, it was my mother who came running out of the kitchen, waving her hands in the air, shouting, and repeating a new word: 'Manure. It's bloody manure.' And on being informed that we were actually jumping into rotting horse poo, reality kicked in. We became aware of the smell and the mess we were in, and the sweet little girl in the once flowered dress began to cry once more. Although like me the boy was not that bothered, needless to say, I never saw either of them again.

The older folk of my lineage were small in height, and in some cases less than 5 feet tall, and I became aware of my own growth rate.

They were deeply set in their ways, and one practice that appeared to be quite widespread was forcing the children to endure a weekly ritual of being dosed with cod liver oil, and a face-squeezing substance called quinine. And thinking that was bad, Sunday nights brought an even worse experience, in the form of a large spoonful of California Syrup of Figs, a liquid potion that tasted absolutely disgusting, but apparently it was good for our bodily functions.

On a positive note, an event worth looking forward to, came around once a year when a visit to the Tower Circus took pride of place. As we entered the arena, the senses were alerted to the smell of animals, the sounds of the audience, and as we took our seats inside the circular rows, a feeling that something exciting was about to happen, stimulated my being. It was a place where different languages could be heard, and as the man in a red jacket wearing a large black hat rolled out his announcements, we all held our breath.

Sighing in unison as gaily costumed people rode bicycles along tight wires, whilst others flew high in the air on swings above tightened safety nets. And as their acts came to an end, loud shouts rang out as funny yet scary-faced clowns on little bikes and cars that blew up, gave way to the red-nosed master.

They called him Charlie Caroli, and his musical silver partner Paul. With laughter all round, the mood suddenly switched to one of anxiety, as the plate spinner played out his act. But it was the erection of high cages, and the red-suited ringmaster who signalled the arrival of lions and tigers. With a snarl and a crack of a whip, they did tricks for the delighted audience.

How grateful we are that those practices are now a thing of the past.

In tune with a scene from the seaside, a family who lived at the back of my grandma's house ran a Punch and Judy show. And on invitation, one day the man gave me a solo performance, a fascinating experience on how it all worked. From his position inside the tent, he had a magical association closely akin with the folk from the house of glass.

My mum's side of the family had arrived on the coast from the distant hills to the east, a place noted for high rainfall that I did not like to visit too often.

Interestingly some houses with outside toilets were amusingly described as having a 'long drop'. My mother's in-laws were funny and had a habit of repeating numerous sayings, like 'They're still hungry when their bellies are full'. I also recall when meeting older people, with nothing in common, they would often ask what I wanted to be when I grew up, and on replying a knight in armour, the conversation usually ended abruptly. In fact, I was always being told that I had too much imagination, and it would get me into trouble one day, a day that was the day, after next.

And as all things must pass, with a degree of sadness on my

part, we moved into a newly built house. It was one of many on an expanding housing estate, the ones that were thrown up to cope with the nation's rising population. At the time they called it the baby boom. In fact, the very same thing is happening once again. For today, like old-time whalers with harpoon in hand, eager men wearing yellow tops, armed with chainsaws, sitting in excavators and small dumper trucks, can be seen attacking the trees and the land with a venomous-like action.

Observer
The last mistle thrush
in the neighbourhood bears witness.
Earth Mother's clock ticks by.
He holds his whistle in readiness, to blow for time.

Des

GYPSIES, SKYLARKS & THE PULL TO THE EAST

The new house, a small thin semi-detached property, had a large rear garden with a brick-built wash-house. Inside, a lounge with an open fireplace, a kitchen with pantry and an adjoining coal shed. The first floor had a bathroom and two bedrooms, I was allocated the smaller one at the front, with linoleum and part carpet laid on the floor; a chimney breast provided some warmth during wintertime. For furniture, a small bedside table, a rosewood wardrobe and with a single bed facing the window, gave rise to the setting sun.

Being a new development, the other young ones with larger families could be seen playing outside, and having left my mystical friends behind, it wasn't long before I too joined in the fun. At the bottom of the avenue, a large caravan park was in the process of being demolished, making way for further housing development. The park site had a dyke border system between the neighbouring farmland, an interesting place where nature flourished. Scores of rabbits lived below the remaining structures of the old buildings, and in the evening time hedgehogs could be seen roaming. As dusk fell, long-eared bats chased their prey, whilst the sound of hooting owls haunted the night. Along with numerous insects and small creatures of the flying kind, not to mention slow-worms and grass snakes, they all managed to live out their lives on the bountiful land. Large numbers of resident birds including hawks and starlings filled the sky, whilst the surrounding fields provided a home for dashing weasels, majestic brown hares, field mice and large toads. Springtime gave rise to the call of the cuckoo, whilst large numbers of ground-nesting birds like the lapwing could be observed. One year I recall some exceptionally large and unknown to me brown geese-like birds staying local for a couple of weeks; they could be found by following their wide tracks through the high grass. They must have been rare, as their arrival gave rise to visiting men with large cameras.

On Saturdays or during the long hot days of the summer holidays, four of us would extend our horizons, setting out on bicycles, visiting places of interest, trainspotting or simply exploring the deeper countryside.

Armed with varying-sized packs of sandwiches, which were usually made up of thin white slices of bread filled with either jam, spam, or a paste of some kind. My favourite was corned beef slices covered in brown sauce, and if we were lucky, pop. One of us may even have brought a bag of plain crisps, and with the added desire to get there, we pushed on. In time we developed a practice of pooling our sandwiches, and in doing so discovered that the food always appeared tastier and seemed to go much further. In fact, at times, we even managed to have some left over for a stop on the return journey home.

From small boys, we had all learnt about the life of Jesus of Nazareth, and whilst putting his miracles aside, we likened our little sharing phenomenon to that of the feeding of the five thousand. For at times when our day-out numbers doubled, those of us with a prepared lunch were willing to pool and share them with those that had little or none. It was noticeable how quickly the barriers that existed between us came down.

Expanding on a youthful finding, with intentional practice, we had cast aside our sense of attachment to 'my' sandwiches. As we lay down our offerings with open hearts, the minds of greed dispersed, we became one with the other boys and our tummies were filled. After lunch, we would sometimes lie down with our backs on the ground, joining the friendly grasshoppers and crickets, and with closed eyes, just listened. In those times wildlife was still in abundance, and through the natural sounds of the countryside came the distinguishing warbling sound of skylarks. Streaky-brown birds with small Mohican-style crests, who lived on the ground and would rise up to great heights, and like tiny helicopters remained in position, by the fluttering of wings. Focusing our eyes, the game was to see who could spot the highest lark in the clear blue sky; the heights they achieved were remarkable, and yet we could still identify the melodic sound of an individual bird, and as all thoughts receded, the lark became us and the land became the sky.

The area around our patch had a farm school for naughty lads, and on the land were numerous freshwater ponds, pits full of water that over time had become havens for wildlife, with coots, moorhen, water voles, frogs and the great crested newt, a favourite of boys, as they resemble mini crocodiles.

And with ample open ground nearer home providing space for the lighting of campfires, the playing of sports, with steam trains and rambling hills all within bike-riding distance, whilst a few pence on the bus took us to the coast, the evenings and the long days and weeks of summertime were never boring.

One thing I did learn from that era was the dangers of certain foods, for when we first moved into the new house, we didn't have a fridge, only a pantry with a cold stone slab. And with that in mind the mothers would generally shop on a daily basis, and after purchase, my mum would wrap the meats and cheeses in greaseproof paper, placing them separately upon the cold slab.

Much to my amusement, Mum would constantly smell the meat, in case it had gone off. At first, I thought she was being silly, until one day after a period of hot weather, a felt pressure change, dark clouds loomed and it became clammy. Mum returned from the kitchen with a package; she asked me to smell the pork, and much to my amazement, it smelt really awful, gone-off.

I was converted to the practice of smelling, and as the chops were quickly dispersed into the dustbin, a lesson learnt, and I gave it much deeper thought. For it made me more aware, and I began to observe the swill men, those characters who regularly came to school to collect and remove the food leftovers, the slops that over time had accumulated in waste bins at the rear of the school canteen. On arrival, the men of the swill would pick up the bins and carry them shoulder-high to a flat back truck, tipping and pouring the stinking contents into larger vessels. Then, whilst engulfed in an indescribably foul stench, they jumped into the cab of the truck and drove off to the next location, before finally taking the full vessels away to feed the pigs. Being a declared pig lover, I found this disgusting practice completely unacceptable, for with my own eyes I had observed pigs living in the woodland at the farm school, where they roamed semi-free, feeding off the ground as nature had intended. Now the pig farmers were keeping them in tightly packed concrete pens, whilst feeding them with rotten human waste. And with a ship or plane journey across to India, pigs can be seen living and foraging through middens, eating excrement, and these practices have all given rise to a belief that pigs are disgusting creatures, the lowest form of life. However, if you turn that around, there is a blessing.

For there is a belief that Buddha Shakyamuni fell violently ill and died of food poisoning from eating a pork dish. And with India having an expanding population approaching 1.5 billion, mostly vegetarians, one can only imagine the consequences if they all ate meat.

Late spring brought the arrival of seasonal visitors, they came in the form of travelling Romanies, Gypsy folk who suddenly appeared in horse-drawn carriages. One of the families set up camp on spare land adjacent to the old caravan site, and apart from the horses it was the colourful clothing and the aura of mystery that drew my attention.

The family consisted of a dark-skinned young man wearing

THE DRUID IN THE GREENHOUSE

boots and trousers, a shirt and waistcoat with a red neck scarf and other accessories. Whilst his lady made home in a long colourful skirt, a red-and-white blouse, head scarf and bracelets. And together with their two small children, they lived a full life within and outside of their vardo. Black and white tethered horses called cobs and with dogs of varying sizes created an invisible boundary, and with a cauldron hanging above an open fire, I was fascinated to discover that there were alternative ways of life available for those that chose to do so. My parents and the other older occupiers of the conforming brick-built houses were not at all impressed, in fact, unhappy with their arrival, and we were told stories of what could happen to young children if they strayed too close to their camp site, especially at night.

Sometimes another Gypsy man appeared on a bike, knocking on the doors of the neighbourhood, he offered to sharpen our kitchen knives and garden shears; most of the male residents eagerly agreed to pay a small fee.

The other side of their arrival brought shawled dark-faced women to our doorsteps, those selling handmade clothes pegs and small bunches of heather, and maybe the occasional rabbit's foot, which was not so lucky for our bob-tailed friends. I kept rabbits as pets, whilst the man next door took great pleasure in informing me that his were for the pot. The young and still scarf-clad housewives of the neighbourhood, whilst half fancying the dark and strong-looking young Gypsy men, feared their women folk, and even took to hiding behind curtains when the Romanies came calling. And if the door was not opened, and a quick peep around the curtain was spotted, then a curse may be cast upon the family doorstep, and so the fear of the unknown no doubt brought ample business to the travelling callers. I found the whole process fascinating, and although being a little fearful, I allowed curiosity to get the better of me.

My daily activities, sometimes deliberate, took me past the small camp, and as familiarisation loosens the shackles of the mind, the sense of fear began to fade. On approach I began to shorten my stride, and the arc around the camp lessened, one of the dogs began to come over to smell me, and the long-roped tethered horses took on a more friendly look. It was about this time that the busy young man of the family began to offer a nod; it was a slow process, but in time the waters of separation began to part. The man started to speak the odd word, until the day came when he pointed and offered me a seat on the bank at the rear of his open fire. I willingly obliged, but with some caution. Communication by tongue was a little difficult, so the movement of hands remained at the forefront. I was offered a hot drink, and although scared of what might be in it, I still accepted his offer, and on doing, the bricks in the wall of long-standing slid down. Sitting higher at the rear of the camp, I observed the man putting wood on the fire, and as his lady cooked from her cauldron, in foreign tongue she gave instructions to her young ones, and yet somehow, I knew what she meant. From my spot I could see right into their wagon, and although exceedingly small, it had a look and a sense of magic, for it fascinated me as to how they all lived in such a small space. But it was the land outside that extended their home, an action that nowadays we may call bifocal, for it was the simplicity of being at one with the whole of nature that brought its rewards.

And with friendship offered, I got to know the man's wife and his children, and each time I passed, smiles and words of kindness were exchanged. As the occasional meet-up became more regular, it was the stimulation of the senses, the drifting smell of food cooked over an open wood fire, their animals, and the growing sense of the freedom to roam, that opened the doors of perception to another way. However, I came from the other side of the tracks, and folk on my side disapproved; people that I didn't even know began shouting 'Gypsy Lover', whilst some of the bigger lads would not miss a chance to be divisive. They informed me that Gypsies were clever, that it was a trap; they were luring me in, and then one day they would put something into my drink, and whilst unconscious, they would tie me up, hold me captive, and I would be taken away to a terrible place, and forced to eat hedgehog.

I never dared tell them that I had already been offered and had eaten the hog of the hedge. But wagging tongues and talk of them not being Christians stirred my mum and dad, and so they too became fearful and concerned for my welfare. Although I believed they were all wrong, out of some feeling of loyalty, and under pressure, I pulled back from my visits to the camp. At first, I would still give a slight nod or a wave as I passed by, but the arc increasingly widened until I eventually made a detour.

As I write, I still feel guilty about ignoring the Romany man; I had disowned him and his family who had been friendly and kind to me. And as the season changed, with the crowing of a cockerel they were gone. On that first morning, upon seeing the empty campsite, I felt ashamed and a coward for not standing up for what I believed in. I promised myself that when they came back next year, I would go and apologise to the man.

I looked out for their vardo, but sadly the colourful family with their unique way of life never returned. Others did arrive in more conventional caravans, but it was not to be, and within a couple of years new building work began and the modern age gobbled up the land.

For me it is a shame that the world of today does not allow for the practice of the old ways, the alternative folk who nowadays get shoved under pylons beside damp motorway bridges, and resort to other ways to simply exist. I would say that I am not particularly a Gypsy lover, just a lover of all, to live and let live, one who holds a belief that there should be a place, a comfortable space, which allows all folk and creatures of this now struggling planet to live out their lives in harmony and peace.

Throughout this period, I had been a member of the Wolf Cubs, an organisation based on the characters created by Rudyard Kipling in his *Jungle Book*, set in the central Indian state of Madhya Pradesh and based on the life of Mowgli, a human boy, who was adopted into the Seoni wolf cub pack. A timeless fascinating tale, it is no coincidence that *The Jungle Book* is still an international box office attraction.

Apart from Mowgli, the other main characters came in the form of Akela the wolf pack leader, Bagheera the black panther, Baloo the bear, Shere Khan the tiger and a python called Kaa who collectively stimulated my imagination.

In our area the Wolf Cub packs of the district held an annual event, a competition, with each pack providing a team that acted out the characters from *The Jungle Book*. We had never previously entered the event, and for past years it had always been won by the same pack, one whose presentation was considered to be outstanding. As the event was being held at their HQ, to say we were the underdogs was putting it mildly.

The competition consisted of individual movements, with two collective main exercises. Akela selected five cubs, and being the senior, I was given the task of leader. For the main event we chose to be Kaa the python, and by linking ourselves together formed the body of the snake. We eagerly took to the practice, and after weeks of dedication and hard work, the day of judgement finally came around. We arrived to find the hall packed full of spectators, and as a small group we sat huddled together on the floor of the room; we watched as other packs displayed their talent. Some were good, others not so, but the home team stood out like true professionals, and in appreciation the audience including our own group leaders were convinced that they would be the outright winners, whilst we were written off as gambolling lambs in a field of mature sheep. But in truth, the five of us remained quietly confident, for there had been occasions during the rehearsals when we all just stopped thinking, and in unison, we felt ourselves being taken over by a force, one that transformed us into the snake Kaa. We knew that if we could achieve and hold that level during the main evening event, then anything could happen.

By the end of the individual and smaller group displays we were still in there holding our own, and as we entered the final stage, we were due to go second to last, following the champions. We sat and watched as they delivered an almost perfect performance, and as the audience belted out their appreciation, the five of us stood up, walked out in unison. As the applause for them died down, we stood in line before the room, and slightly bowed our heads, amazingly we had never done or even discussed that in practice.

As we moved in line at the side of the stage, turning we arched our backs, and with heads facing downwards, stretched out our arms and linked with the one in front. Being the head of the great snake, with arms outstretched and hands touching in prayer-like position, we stood ready. Upon hearing the sound to commence, whilst moving on the spot in motion with body and tail, we set off on the same leg, and our performance began.

As we moved through the early stages of the set, I still recall a voice from behind saying, 'It's happening, it's happening,' and on stepping through a door of pure light, we danced and weaved our way into a magical trance, a timeless space, where only Kaa the snake existed.

And as the finale approached, I had the task of delivering words spoken, now lying snake-like on the floor, and with only my head raised, I announced, 'Shere Khan is dead. Shere Khan is dead. Shere Khan is dead,' and on slipping down over the tail of the body, the sound of silence filled the jungle auditorium. I was completely gone, just a snake lying down, but we were slowly brought back to human form by the sound of the exuberant audience who had obviously appreciated our performance. As we rose in a post-trance state, we knew we had done it. On having re-joined the audience we awaited the judge's decision, and against all the odds we won the competition. We took to the stage to receive the applause, but for us the material prize didn't really matter. For what we had all learnt and taken away from the experience was the realisation of the power of the union of body and mind, and later in life, that of the shapeshifter.

I cannot recall who the other lads were, and I do wonder what became of them. It was around the same time that I was exposed to my first serious non-ordinary experience, and it happened whilst asleep in my bedroom.

Sometime during the night, I was awakened by the sound of strange music, followed by a loud shuffling sound, and on opening my eyes, I was shocked to see four figures, standing in a row at the bottom of my bed. They were over 5 feet in height and had large colourful scary-looking heads. My immediate thoughts were that I was dreaming but on confirmation that I was awake, my thoughts quickly changed to that of my friends messing about. It would have been brilliant if that was the case, but unfortunately, I ruled that one out. The figure on the left of the row, a male, appeared to be the leader, and as he gestured with his right arm, the others swayed, and with a humming-like sound, they began to slightly move around. He then began

THE DRUID IN THE GREENHOUSE

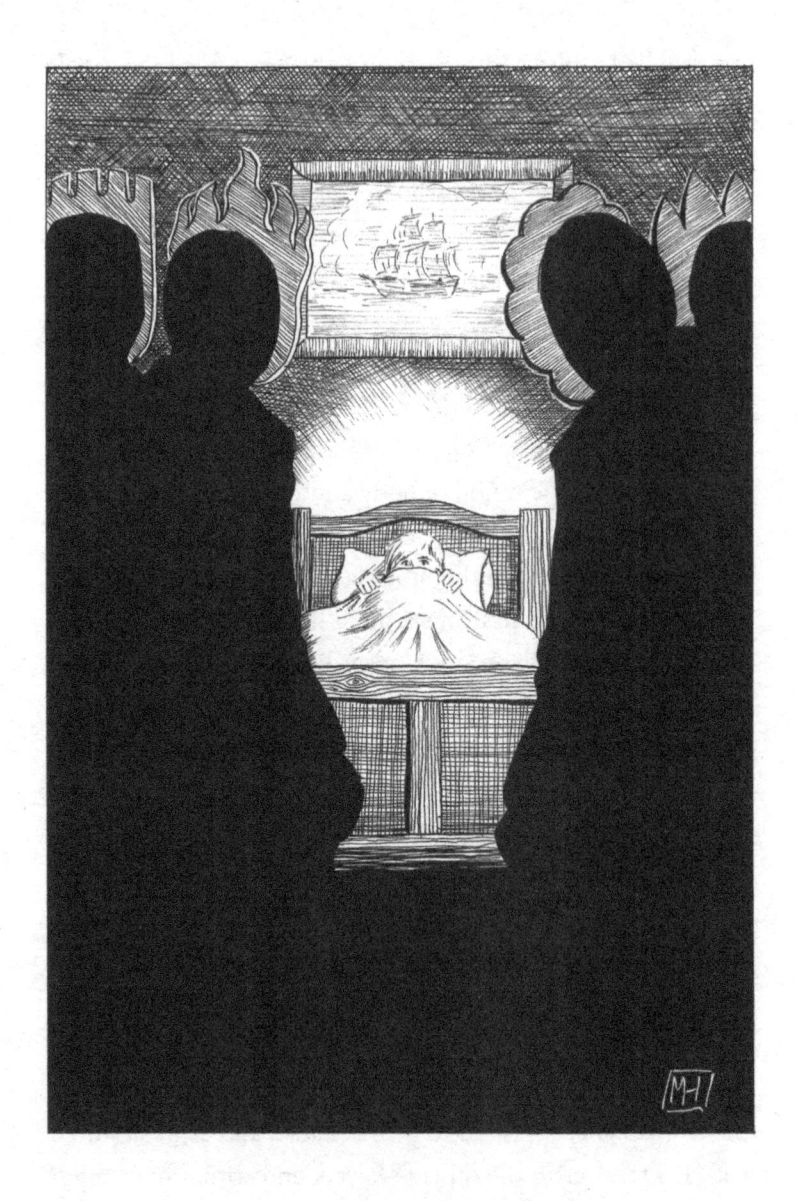

Otherworldly Visitors – In the Bedroom

speaking to me in a manner that I did not understand, and with extreme trepidation I dived down below the bedding.

Whilst lying their cocooned in a hot and breathless state, I could still hear them, and on taking a quick peep, they remained right there, still in a line at the end of the bed. Eventually, for what seemed like an age, I heard the shuffling sound, and after waiting a while longer, took another peep to confirm they had gone. As I sat up in bed pondering, I really had no idea what it had all been about, I knew I could not tell anyone, at a push my mum, but she would just say that I had been having a nightmare. Alarmingly, the visits became a regular happening, the act of being awakened in the night made me fearful of falling asleep. That was until one evening whilst sat up in bed reading, I heard the now familiar sound of strange music, but this time I was totally awake, and that realisation shook me to the core. The four figures came shuffling into the room from the gap between the wardrobe and the front wall, and like previous times they stood facing me at the end of the bed whilst motioning and speaking to me in strange tongues. I did not understand why they had come to my room, what did they want from me? I wished they would tell me, but they just continued with the same action, and once again dived below the sheets and wished they would go away.

I decided to inform my mother. She listened and then told me to stop being silly, as it was just a nightmare, I had expected her to say that, but what else could she say about the unexplainable. The appearance of the people with huge horrendous faces continued, and then suddenly their visits ceased and normality returned. But after a break of a few weeks, they appeared once more, and in time, I became less scared, I began to speak back to them, but they seemed programmed and continued to repeat the same motions.

Did they want me to go somewhere with them? I had thought about that and may well have been willing to do so, but it was the not knowing that was definitely having an effect on me.

Can you imagine being asked each morning if you had a good night's sleep? And being at school, taking lessons in various subjects, when all I really wanted to learn about was where the four men with large heads came from and what they wanted of me?

Eventually one evening and with some regret, I knelt down and prayed for them to stop coming to my bedroom, and they never visited me again. I never did have any idea as to why they came and what they wanted from me, but what I had learnt was the power of prayer.

All appeared to return to normal once more, until one night whilst watching a variety television programme with my parents, a man came on stage, and whilst changing hats delivered a poem, which commenced:

There is a one-eyed yellow idol to the north of Kathmandu,
There's a little marble cross below the town.
There's a broken-hearted woman tends the grave of Mad Carew,
And the Yellow God forever gazes down.

J Milton Hayes

On hearing those spoken words, I was rocked, taken aback, as it connected with the four figures who had visited my room, it resonated from deep within my young being. As I sat there in the room with my parents, I had to secretly hold on tight, as I slipped away into a trance-like state. Bearing in mind that as a boy in 1960, apart from *The Jungle Book,* I had no outside contact with anything remotely connected to the East of this planet. But what it did, was open me, illuminate my being, and with a strong desire to learn, the seeds of the seeker were sown.

SATANIC MILLS AND THE MAHATMA

On two or three occasions each year, I would accompany my mum and aunt to visit our relatives in the mill towns of East Lancashire. Coming from a vibrant seaside town, it was an early reality check, for it was an area that I would later hear described as having dark satanic mills.

However, this time was a little different, for we intended to stay over, and arriving in the middle of the afternoon, with our hosts still at work, we had no means of entry, so we walked up to the mill to collect the house keys.

Whilst climbing a steep cobbled street, you know the ones, those hemmed in on all sides by rows of terraced houses, we approached a side street, and like two trolley buses taking a bend in a busy town centre, we brushed past a group of interestingly dressed young women. I was amazed, as the ladies were all wearing brightly coloured long garments, bracelets, jewellery with rings in their noses; they were of the like that I had never seen before.

Overcome by fascination, I just stood in the middle of the

street pointing and shouting for my mum and aunt to look; the ladies of colour responded with waving hands and wide smiles, whilst my mother apologised for my behaviour once again. I was informed that they were from Pakistan and had come to this country to work in the cotton mills; in fact, the very same mill that we were actually walking too. But I still didn't understand why such colourful people would ever want to come here in the first place. On arrival at the mill, we passed through a side entrance, where we met a lady, my aunt knew; she gave us permission to go in and get the keys. We proceeded through two large swing doors, and entered a huge deafening place, full of machines, moving parts, the noise level was so loud, the workers had to use sign language.

However, we were enthusiastically welcomed and given the key to my other aunt's front door. Back then people had different values from those of today, for during and after the war, people had become displaced, families were torn apart, there were many orphans, and folk took children in and brought them up as if they were their own. Religion had a power of influence, and like resistance groups in wartime, families feared that others may discover their secrets, and as the sins of the family followed the daughter, just as today, many things went on behind drawn curtains.

I recall it was a small, terraced house, with steep stairs set behind a door in the front room wall. Later, we were all sat around the table, eating ample portions of homemade cakes, all washed down with umpteen cups of freshly brewed tea, creating a scene a tad like 'Bettys of Harrogate' without the trimmings.

It all must have had an effect, for the other auntie, the one who lived in the house, lit the candle of encouragement, my uncle instantly responded by jumping up and opening the chimney breast cupboard. And in doing, activated a rite of ceremony: the rolling out of the family photo album. Actually, they were an assortment of biscuit tins that amazingly contained a collection of old black and white photographs, those of my ancestors on my mother's side of the family. And as a young Dalai Lama explores his own past-life treasures, I was guided through a timeline of grandads, and uniformed uncles, the ones who had enthusiastically marched off to war, some never to return. There were great-aunts dressed as nurses, cousins in costumes during religious and national events, and even a picture of my young mother as a land girl, stood in front of her 1930s-built truck.

On placing my hand over the China teacup, offerings of ginger beer and dandelion and burdock were freely accepted. I had enjoyed seeing the old family pics, but it was a larger photograph that drew my attention.

On closer inspection, it revealed a scene outside a large building; at the centre stood a group of exuberant local female mill workers, and amongst them a man who appeared quite different, dressed inappropriately for the climate of the region. He stood there smiling, wrapped in a white loin cloth, with only sandals on his feet, and wearing distinguished round spectacles.

I felt instantly drawn to his presence. His name was Mahatma Gandhi, and my uncle eagerly told me the story of the little Indian man, who in the early 1930s had come over to England. And when visiting this area, he had explained to the local mill workers that the cotton they were using had been grown in India. And the people of India under British rule were not allowed to manufacture their own products, and they had to purchase more expensive foreign-made goods. He asked the mill workers for their support, and amazingly they gave it.

His story stimulated me, and I later learnt how this man of small physical proportions had overcome the might of the British Empire. He had observed their weakness, defeating them by the philosophy of ahimsa, the action of non-violence, the complete absence of ill will against them.

My interest in Gandhi the Father of India flowed with me through life and many years later during a visit to Delhi, I consciously stood inside a sparse room, and before me his spinning wheel, a space where his famous round spectacles lay on a nearby desk. Gandhi the Mahatma, who once stated that he travelled third class on a train, because there was not a fourth.

As a boy I had divided feelings for animals, the nicer-looking ones like the birds, voles, hares, bees, frogs, and newts I loved, and viewed them as friends. Yet not so the flying beetles, the flies, and especially the wasps those free stingers, who we saw as the enemy.

One afternoon I set out on a solo 40-minute bike ride, and on arrival at a farmyard was granted permission to fish, and with bag over my shoulder and rod in hand, I hiked across a couple of fields to my favourite pond. A spot of sheer beauty away from the roads, buildings and overhead power lines, a sacred place, a realm of pure nature, where I could simply immerse myself in the pursuit of catching my favourite fish, the splendid crucian carp. The L-shaped pool had a lovely tree-lined setting full of reeds, water lilies and a host of marginal plants, a place where the larger species of fish chose to live.

Yet the far bank was my chosen spot to fish that day, but on arrival I discovered that it had recently become more difficult to gain access, for the farmer had decided to use the steep bank for the disposal of his cut-down foliage. Having selected a route of passage, and with bag and rod in hand I overcame the tricky climb down, and on setting up my tackle, cast my baited hook into the tranquil water. The setting was so peaceful, and with the fish feeding from the off, all was well. A pair of large blue emperor dragonflies arrived on the scene, and like tiny WWI biplanes, they buzzed around below the leaved branches of the overhanging trees. Then suddenly I became a target, and as the larger of the two flew straight at me, I flapped my hands to fend it off, but it repeated its actions, and I became frightened. I reacted by picking up my metal rod rest, and lashing out, I delivered a blow, a fatal one that sent the creature into a spinning motion, and as it fell down upon the still water, it laid on its back motionless.

The remaining one of the pair instantly responded, flying down, and hovering above the body of its dead partner, and as it became disturbingly clear, I could only sit there staring, absorbing the suffering that my action had created.

As the whole of the pond fell silent, Mother Nature turned towards me, and shook her head in dismay. For I realised that I had just shattered the window of a perfect place, a small place where everything was incredibly beautiful, until this little human boy, whom they had come to trust, had come along, and spoilt everything. And as the brightness of the day turned to that of dark grey, I quickly packed up my gear and left for home. For some it would have been just an action, a method of removing an annoying dragonfly, but for me it ran much deeper. Through a moment of inner fear, I had allowed myself to respond in a manner that had left me with a feeling that I had just punctured a hole through the framework of existence, and that was something I would have to live with. I did go back on a couple of occasions, but it was not the same, the magic was missing, my membership had been withdrawn.

The memory of my actions on that day stayed with me, as they still do to this day, it had been an unpleasant experience, one created by my own cowardly action. I felt the guilt, the shame, and had rightly received an otherworldly telling-off, and so the positive I took away was a spiritual one. I realised long ago that the greatest experiences involving nature come about when a person is on their own, even a simple thing like rising around dawn. Stepping outside before the start-up of traffic, when the early morning chi is most active, the universe feels so welcoming, and you do not understand why everyone else is still in bed.

SUNNY DAYS

In times past, the daughter became her mother and the son his father.

On Monday mornings, the men went off to work, and for the young housewife, it was washday, a labour-intensive chore that even with the aid of boilers, a mangle and some torturous-looking tools could actually take all day. And on the mention of torturous tools, there was one word that terrified all children, a word that on hearing, brought out the sweats, in fact sheer terror, a place they called the school dentist.

In those days they were obsessed with the action of extracting teeth.

And on the dawn of the day of the appointment, and with half a mind to run away, I left home accompanied by Mum; it commenced with a bus journey, followed by a long walk up a hill, and it was on that last leg that we became exposed to telltale signs. Recent pools and stains of red vomit could be spotted at kerb sides and on the pavements by walled gardens, noticeably increasing in volume as we approached the House of Terror. The dental building was located at the top of the hill facing a school playground, and as we turned to walk the final leg of the journey, bent figures of young children with mums in attendance could be seen leaning against walls, and amongst hedgerows, retching and vomiting blood and bile, for they had been gassed.

Yet the front of the building had a pleasant appearance, but regulars would not be fooled; access was gained along a bush-lined path, and on arrival we opened the doors of entry. It was a large open room, with rows of seats laid out on either side of a central aisle that led to the registration desk, and at the rear of the desk sat a large man, and before him, a brass bell with wooden handle.

Having registered, the boys and girls were sent to separate sides of the aisle. At this point of the proceeding's words could not describe the fear that gripped those poor young souls. On registering and taking our seats I glanced around the room at my fellow captives; some shuffled with edginess, whilst others closed down, cocooned in fear, as they awaited the dreaded call. If it was a first visit, then the stories told haunted you. However, if it was a return visit, as in my case, then you were fully conscious of the horrors that awaited the call of your name. Then it happened, and as the trap door beneath your feet partially opened, the man at the registration desk rose up, and on the placement of a black cloth, picked up and rang the hand bell. It was a reverberating sound, which caught the immediate attention of the entire room, and as the young ones waited for the vibrations to wane, I glanced around. It seemed like an age before a name was called, and if it wasn't familiar, then a sigh of relief followed, but it was only a brief stay of execution. I did think about running, but where would I go? Within no time at all, the desk man rose once more, and no matter how many poor souls were awaiting sentence, I always knew when it was my turn. True to form the bell rang, and my full name was called. I rose to my feet, and all alone took the long walk past the bell-ringer, only to be met by a stern-looking man and a woman who escorted me down a long side corridor.

On the way I could hear the groans and shrieks of young children in distress, those sights and sounds that people of the modern age would have difficulty in recognising. We reached the last room on the left, and on entry I was met by a half-circle of adults; they were dressed in white coats and wore false smiles.

In the centre of the room stood a drilling machine, with an expanding arm that was powered by pulleys and thick webbed fan belts, and below a large light was a reclining leather seat, with footplate and headrest. Before climbing into the chair, I was told to undo all the buttons on my short trousers, although I never knew why, I heard the door close behind me. Large hands slid me back, a piece of something hard was inserted into my small mouth, and with many hands at work, a rubber-smelling mask was inserted over my face, I was instructed to take in deep breaths. Poisonous gas filled my young lungs, the voices of the white coats began to distort, the mask became a part of my face that extended upwards. As the gas took over, I became a rubber rope that was attached to the centre of the ceiling, and I started to slowly swirl in a widdershins direction.

As the swirling motion increased in speed, I began to fly around the room, rising above the equipment, whilst consciously fretting that I might hit something. At the height of the exercise, the head was forced to rock, and then like nearing of the end of a ride at the fun fair of fear, the motion started to slow down, and once again the fear of hitting the machines returned. Distorted voices could be heard, as I came back down to land once more into the dreaded chair. Rough hands pulled the rubber wedge and blood-soaked swabs from my twisted mouth; I could make out the staring faces, who with handed gestures encouraged me to stand. And with falling trousers around weakened knees, two white coats dragged me staggering into an adjoining room, lined with a row of small sinks. I still recall another child, a small girl struggling to stand up as she splatted the white porcelain with her own blood and vomit. Of course, compassion had not yet been invented, but I felt for the young thing; I attempted to go to her aid, only to be rebuked by a white coat in attendance. But with the churning of the stomach, it was my turn to arch over the tiny sink, and I too became helpless.

After a time, I became a little more aware of the senses, the door to the room opened and a boy came staggering in. With the immediate effects of the gas starting to wear off, I was ushered through a side exit door, and with the finesse of a hard-core drunk leaving an all-night boozing session, I stepped out into the bright daylight. On realising which way to turn, a squinted glance revealed the shimmering shape of my mother who stood waiting anxiously at the end of the path to freedom.

But the ordeal was not over, for as we turned left to go down the hill, I started to vomit once more, and as the new arriving children watched on, we caught up with the young girl and her distraught mother, and as our two mums exchanged opinions of disgust, we simply hung on in there.

Imagine if we had instantly become childhood sweethearts, and later in life were asked where we first met, and what we then had in common.

It was a barbaric and cold experience played out at a time when the adults were hardier than those of today. In fact, my friends and I likened it to the happenings inside the dungeons of a medieval castle. But it had much in common with the senior school I attended, where corporal punishment was keenly dished out, on a daily basis.

Looking back, I always had the same gas induced dream, and on comparing the experience with other children, I discovered that interestingly they had different effects from the gas. After a week the mouth started to heal, but the psychological damage remained, and like all the other children and their mothers, we continued to live in fear of the drop of the dreaded letter.

Thankfully, that was to be the last time I ever visited the bell-ringer's domain. Our world moved on, compassion came in, Victorianism died out, gas was replaced with a novocaine injection, and my future dental work was conducted by a gentleman at a standard practice.

FREE-FALLING AND THE WICKER MAN

In a time before global warming, whilst out on a car drive with my father and uncle, we crossed over a large newly constructed road bridge. I was informed that it was a new section of the M6 motorway, and on completion, motorists would be able to drive from Birmingham to Carlisle without stopping.

My uncle, the eldest brother, saw that it would allow the masses to come and spoil our secret hideaways and beauty spots, whilst my father was not so sure, as he could see the opportunity for long-distance travel. Whereas being the younger one, I saw it as a happening, it would cut hours off congested A-road journeys to the mountains and forests of the Lake District, Scotland, and North Wales.

It appeared natural that many of the older generation had a dislike for change, and in doing so, criticised the young for their modern views and opinions.

People often become attached to their ways, their belief systems. However, in some cases they may well be correct, and like all things, the answer usually lies in accepting a sensible balance. On a stroll in the park, you may catch sight of grandparents simply enjoying the moment watching their grandchildren excitedly feeding the ducks. And as a young girl cruises by on an electric skateboard, you may well hear one say, 'Well, it's their time now, love.'

As the green shoots of the flowers of the 1960s pushed skywards, I took the leap from Wolf Cub to Boy Scout, an action that opened the door to an exciting new world. For being a scout in uniform meant I could legally carry a sheath knife, and lo and behold a staff. Having learnt about map-reading with a compass, my scope for adventure expanded, and after being introduced to long hikes across valleys, mountains, and moorland, it was the preparing of camp, a night shelter, bivouacking against trees and stone walls, that stimulated my imagination. The occasional luxury of cooking a freshly caught brown trout over the embers of an open fire, a dish that complemented the standard fare of tins of baked beans and London grill. Learning how to make dough dampers, that when cooked over a hot stone, sliced, and filled with butter and jam, were simply delicious. The world of the Boy Scout had the motto 'Be Prepared', a statement bearing power, but Be Prepared for what? 'For life, son, for Life,' came a stern reply from the ex-military scout leader. We were taught survival skills, including planning and reconnaissance. Prior to setting off on long hikes and wild camps we understood the need to keep matches dry, and to carry spare batteries for the cumbersome torch, spare boot laces or string, and a first aid kit. I even learnt how to darn a hole in a woollen sock.

Long before mobiles, two young teenagers out in the wilds,

whether in steep wooded valleys, or on a misty mountain ridge, survival by using the senses, the smells, an awareness to change, the sight of approaching dark clouds, the feel of a subtle pressure or wind direction. Remaining vigilant, reading nature, the sounds of animal, a friendly human or maybe a foe.

Just being aware of your own personal safety, when worsening icy conditions call for single-pointed mindfulness with every step. The phrase 'Be Prepared' was etched into my being. Yet it was not just about the physical, but how one also reacts to a verbal attack, statements, phrases delivered with harmful intentions, the way we respond to bad news, and an over-reaction to the good.

It was a midsummer day in the early 1960s, when a large party of scouting people boarded a Liverpool steamer, a four-hour crossing to the ancient kingdom of the Isle of Man. On arrival our spirits were high, forming chains to carry and load our equipment onto the awaiting buses, and once aboard, we set off in a northerly direction. On arrival at the campsite, we split into separate groups, my troop choosing to pitch our tents on the flat ridge of a hill, and with views overlooking a river bottomed tree-lined valley, all felt good.

As it turned out, it rained constantly for most of the time, and for anyone that has experienced those conditions whilst living under canvas miles away from anywhere, at times it can be quite challenging.

However, I took two frames of experience from the trip.

It was a mid-afternoon after the rain had ceased, when four of us decided to take leave of the camp to explore, to see what the view of our site looked like from the ridge on the opposite side of the valley.

Setting off from the rear of our tents we scrambled down the side of the hill, and on reaching the stony valley bottom, managed to find the safest route across the swollen river. After a bit of squelching around, we set off to climb up the tree-lined slope, on reaching the top we discovered it was very rocky with large boulders deposited from an age long ago. After exploring the immediate area, we settled down amongst the shaded boulders for a leisurely drink and a snack. But as the other side of the valley always looks more appealing, being a committed tree climber, I decided to ascend the largest of the trees.

Two of the lads were content to stay on the ground, whilst the other one, a future principal, climbed the same tree as me, but he decided to perch himself out across a lower branch, and with his legs dangling continued in conversation with the lads below. A good way up the tree I got the first view of our camp site, followed by a sudden desire to climb to the very top, and with fear nowhere to be found, I had an uncontrollable urge to continue skywards. Rising higher and higher through the greenery until I could no longer make out the ground below me, I was almost there, then suddenly I heard a crack, and instantly entered the sensation of falling. Time as we know it ceased to exist, I was aware of facing the trunk, and the colour of brown, flashes of branches passed by me, from my left I caught a glimpse, the form of a presence, and an awareness of a motion that turned me completely around to face outwards.

Free-falling, I could see the rocky ground and the sight of

a figure on a branch below me, I felt and allowed myself to be guided further out and away from the trunk of the huge tree. And on being aligned, like a crane lowering a steel structure into position, I dropped into place, sitting upright with my legs around the neck and across the shoulders of the future headmaster.

He knew nothing of my fall, he was hurt and shouted at me for jumping on him, and as we both swayed precariously like an untrained high-wire act at the circus, the two other lads responded by coming to our rescue, and after a few more hair-raising minutes, we manage to unlock and climb back down onto the boulder-strewn ground once more. They were all in shock, I was something different, as the realisation that a divine intervention had brought about a miraculous landing, for I was in no doubt at all that I would have died aged 13. In conclusion, I had responded to a sudden desire to rise to touch the top, a pinnacle, a summit where nothing existed below me, and on coming down I did not panic, stayed within myself, allowing a greater force to assist me in the closure of the experience. The future principal was temporarily injured, I was physically fine, and we all laughed it off as we made our way back down the side of the valley. Another wetting as we crossed the river, before reaching the safety of our camp site. After a life-changing or potentially life-ending experience, we tend to consciously replay the incident over and over again, but oddly, I was more overcome by a sense of wonder. Some would say what a load of rubbish, whilst others would feel that I had been saved by my guardian angel, as it was not the time or the place for me to go. Needless to say, I resisted the urge to try and touch a pinnacle, in fact my desire to climb trees also receded. During the days at the summer camp a lot of the time was spent on basic living, going to river, and returning with full buckets of water, collecting kindling and the correct wood for burning, lighting fires, cooking, and washing up, keeping the shared tents and the site tidy, not to mention emptying latrines and personal hygiene. Most evenings were spent sat around a large open fire, and I recall the occasion when the scout leaders collectively stated that we should all enjoy the camp, as we will grow up to view it as the best time of our lives.

The leaders must have given that some thought, but for me they had made a judgement based on their lifetime experiences, as we were a different generation adapting to a different world. As older folk tend to look back at the glorified high points of their lives, so too the young look forward to the future, to live the dream of material gains.

And as Mrs Barn Owl watched on from the opening in a nearby tree, she whispered to her owlets, 'They can only ever live in the present moment, as the other two do not exist.' Back then we had yet to experience the fullness of life, yet we were free spirits, full of adventure, with minds of positivity.

Towards the end of the second week the rain finally eased off, and with a day out arranged, we took a bus journey down to the south of the island, and whilst going over Fairy Bridge we were encouraged to shout 'Good Morning' to the fae folk, an action I found most inspiring.

Having reached our planned destination, the party split

into smaller groups, and with a plan to meet up later in the day, we went our separate ways.

Some of our party, me included, made our way to visit the island's Witch Museum, and on entry there was plenty of banter, along with some scepticism that was nicely wrapped up inside a veil of fear.

As we wandered around the museum, I took time to peer into the cabinets whilst gazing at stands and tables bearing the objects on display.

I was fascinated, and after some time browsing, I realised I was alone in the room, and on venturing out into the rear courtyard, found the rest of my small party, acting strangely. For they had tucked themselves up inside a corner of the yard, and to my mind's eye, they resembled a small herd of cattle stood waiting at a farm gate for milking.

On approaching, I became aware that they were timidly looking towards something, and on turning I observed a long-white-haired bearded gentleman, who stood alone in the centre of the gardened area.

I was then informed that he was a witch, wow, a real witch, well that was it for me, and much to the surprise of my group, I confidently walked across the yard to the distinguished-looking man, and on gazing from close quarters he appeared to be troubled. But without need for ceremony, and without further ado: 'Excuse me, sir. Are you a witch?'

The smallish gentlemen turned to me, and with eyes showing signs of a soul of deep searching, simply replied, 'Yes, I am,' before offering me a wry smile.

For me that was a real wow moment, goodbye Hansel, and Gretel, I had just met a real witch. But I came away from the experience bearing some feeling for him, in fact, unbeknown to me at the time, he was a fellow Lancastrian, and a prominent Wiccan in the name of Gerald Gardner. A man who was highly regarded and seen as the 'Father of Modern Witchcraft'. On the way out I purchased a card bearing his image, one that I still have stored away in a tin to this day.

On arriving back home from camp, it was not long before we returned to school, where the curriculum included a weekly Religious Knowledge class.

As I recall we only ever discussed Christianity, but I liked the teacher and enjoyed his lessons. However, one day he asked the class what we thought were the main issues behind wars and the conflicts of the planet.

Instinctively raising my hand, I said, 'Religion, sir.' Well, his face was a picture, my answer did not go down well, and after a speech, he basically stated that religion stopped conflicts and wars, not started them. I took his comment with some surprise, and my opinion remains the same, as unfortunately it can and does create division.

Just prior to the school's Christmas shutdown, we had a few events to attend, one being the Christmas carol service, held at the local parish church, and much to my surprise, I was chosen as the pupil who would read out a passage from the Bible. Having accepted the task and attended practice sessions the day of the event drew closer, we moved to the parish church for final rehearsals. It was a large building with many rows of wooden pews, in fact, the church was famous for two of its chairs, constructed from timber salvaged from the local beach wreckage of Nelson's flagship, the *Foudroyant*, a wreck that is still visible to this day.

The day of the Christmas carol service came around, and the place was packed with pupils and parents including my proud mum, on entry I took my seat on the front row below the pulpit. With a squelch of breath, the pipe organ came to life, the choir entered, and like a scene from a movie, the sounds of Christmas present reverberated around the high walls and ceiling of the now energised building. After an introduction and another couple of carols the vicar made his way to the pulpit and we settled down into our seats for his festive time sermon. Around twenty minutes later, and with a smile at the congregation the vicar closed his book, looked down and gave me the nod.

I stood up and approached the raised pulpit and waited for the vicar to descend the spiral staircase. He was a hard act to follow, I was aware of the change of atmosphere around me, and with an air of anticipation I gave a nodding smile to the vicar, and ascended. On arrival in the pulpit, and with a slightly nervous foot shuffle, I placed my book upon the lectern, and looking up, the sight of a mass of faces, hundreds of people all staring directly at me. An inner instruction informed me to smile back, and with a conscious intake of breath a feeling of calmness emerged from within, and on turning to the first lines, I commenced my delivery. It was quite a long one, and once again, time took a back seat, and I just went with the flow.

I was confident and regularly glanced up at the sea of heads before me, and on reaching the end, looked around with a smile, bowed my head and said thank you to the congregation, closed the book, and on reaching the steps, I received a welcome applause.

But this was not the end of my churchly experiences, and although I never really knew how or why, I just followed the path of life's intention. One that found me, along with another couple of scout mates recruited into the role of altar boys at my local church, a high one, so I was informed.

It was not something I had ever had a passion for, yet I felt comfortable with a knowing that the knowledge gained by the experience would be beneficial in the long term, so I simply followed my instinct. After completing a period of training, my duties took me to attending a main Sunday service and one early weekday morning communion. I had been an altar boy for around six months when early one weekday morning whilst dressed in red with an outer white smock and carrying a large church stick candle, with flickering flame, I followed the vicar out from the vestry. At that time of the day, unless someone had recently died, there was only ever one regular lady in attendance, and she always sat in the same spot on the front pew. I took a kneeling position on a lower step to the left of the Anglican priest, and as he continued with the service, I felt compelled to stare upwards and towards the hanging image of Jesus of Nazareth.

In doing, I experienced an illumination, pictures of images and messages came in to play, followed by the feeling of an inner reshuffle of my disorderly pack. It was a realisation of enormity that had been bestowed upon me, a map for a path, which put me on a course, to become a spiritual seeker. But what do I seek?

'You must go and seek the truth, like Gandhi did,' said the pipe-smoking Caterpillar from Barnsley

POP SONGS AND THE TURNING TO THE EAST

As the periodic motion of the pendulum depends upon the length of a piece of string, the cultural revolution of the swinging sixties began to accelerate.

Young British musicians who had grown up under the influence of American blues artists transcended cover versions, became songwriters and created their own new sounds.

Pirates had returned to our seas once more, but the clash of the cutlass had been overcome by the sounds of rotating vinyl. However, the ethos was similar or even the same. The strength of the blowing winds of change had not embraced the whole of suburbia, but my weekends were certainly becoming more eventful.

One Saturday morning in the summer of 1964, I headed out into town, stopping off for supplies at a local tuck shop before moving on to the Odeon Cinema, a place now famously recognised as Funny Girls! Being a punctual-minded person, I arrived at the venue a little early, and taking my place at the bottom of the front entrance steps, dipped a hand inside my pocket, slid out a boiled lollypop, and without much effort,

THE DRUID IN THE GREENHOUSE

slipped it into the side of my mouth. I had arranged to meet up with some school mates, and with the arrival of more enthusiastic young people, the atmosphere was starting to build up. But I became distracted, when I was drawn to respond to an inner tug (a something that was becoming more frequent) whilst scanning the horizon, I noticed that across the road outside a well-known coffee bar stood a group of five smartly American style dressed -individuals.

There were three men wearing long coats and Fedora/Trilby hats, two held large cameras, and they were locked in conversation with a pair of extremely attractive, smartly dressed women. Although the movement of town centre traffic prevented a clear view, I was aware that the group were looking and pointing in my direction. It was then that one of the men, accompanied by the two ladies, crossed the road, and took up a position on the pavement by the cinema steps. Then, as if a wet sponge were squeezed over my head, the film-star-looking lady of the two came up the steps towards me, and with a smile straight out of Hollywood politely asked if she could have a word. 'Yes please' was no doubt my reply, and as a large gathering crowd looked on, she explained that they were newspaper reporters and wished to take up a few minutes of my time. 'Not a problem, honey.' As it turned out they were covering the big news story about a young Jamaican girl called Millie Small, whose ska-influenced song, 'My Boy Lollipop', had just reached number two in the British music charts, and in an instant the scene changed. The two camera-bearing men were waved over, and the ladies began to rearrange my appearance, even combing my hair, and as a central spot on the cinema steps was cleared, I was ushered in to position.

I was now in my element, in fact, an aspiring young Bond, and as passers-by stopped to view, even the traffic slowed down. And as the photo-shoot session began, my new film-star girlfriend arranged the style of my poses, and between the resetting sounds and the flashing of cameras, I looked on with lolly in mouth. After numerous shots the photo session ended, my details were taken, the reporters gave their appreciation, the ladies waved goodbye, and we slipped back into our separate lives. As the crowd started to disperse my mates appeared with smiling faces, asking if I was going to be in a movie. Well unfortunately not, but I did feel a bit aggrieved, when a decade later, the American actor Telly Savalas stole my act and became the famous lollypop-licking detective, Kojak.

But I did have fame for a day when my picture appeared on the front pages of the press below the headline 'My Boy Lollipop' and the unfolding story of Millie Small, the young Jamaican girl who had stolen the hearts of the nation. My mum was thrilled, and school friends gave me new nicknames in the form of Lolly Head, but I considered that to be fair game.

The 1960s continued to boom, and with plenty of jobs available, it was the first time that teenagers had money in their pockets and purses, and with the added attraction of living in a holiday town, it provided ample opportunities to earn extra cash. Up until then, and apart from Millie of course, for me the music scene had been silly, a regurgitation of headwear, with only the fading signal of radio Luxembourg providing a beacon of light. But all that changed with the arrival of *Caroline,* a radio ship anchored about 60 nautical miles away in the Irish Sea. And with DJs providing a continuous catalogue of sounds, it was through our crystal-clear transistor radios that a new wave of freshness washed over us. The 1950s Teddy boys were now competing with Beatniks, Mods and Rockers, and as stems of flower power rose, came the changing shape of design, LP covers, models, clothing, photographic art and swinging cane furniture. Hire purchase was freely available, and with money for a deposit, the potential to purchase scooters, motor bikes and cars opened the gates to the field of adventure, and with the added arrival of the contraceptive pill, in came the freedom of choice.

But there was another ingredient that awaited the simmering brew, and that came from the dark corridors of the NHS, when their actions inadvertently pushed the doors of the establishment wide open. By now the young housewives of the baby boom years had obtained automatic washing machines, and having slipped off their head scarfs and shortened their skirts, had started to struggle with mental disorders. And the game plan from the pharmaceutical companies and the doctors of the health service was to prescribe them with medication. This was brought to the forefront by Mick Jagger the front man of the Rolling Stones, with their song 'Mother's Little Helper', an observation about a housewife who abuses her prescription drugs. Those potions of tonics, stimulants, tranquilisers, and the ones that put you to sleep, which when mixed with the weekend's boozy sessions, gave rise to interesting results. It became common for the outgoing young of the gender, to ask each other what their mothers were on. And as the nation's bathroom cabinets were gently opened, the practice slipped undetected into modern youth culture. As the decade progressed and much to the displeasure of parents and the establishment who had previously gone along with the early mop-head Beatles, the arrival of Sergeant Pepper, Pink Floyd, and psychedelia became more than a step too far. When a small group of British musicians travelled to distant places, like Rishikesh in northern India, they returned with speckles of knowledge and tales of mysticism that influenced other young folk to follow their path. And on return, bangles, beads, and various forms of resin, and with a growing acceptance of Caribbean culture, the final influencer came from America, when organic and laboratory-created hallucinogens arrived on our shores.

With the flick of a table lighter in a time of boom came entrepreneurs and the emergence of outdoor music events, and non-alcohol related all-night dance clubs, that today we call raves. A phenomenon of the early to mid-1960s came in the form of an article of clothing called bell bottoms, ex-navy styled trousers that had little bells sewn into them. And in no time at all, it went mainstream. Business-minded people trawled the nations haberdashery stalls and pet shops in search of multicoloured ribbons and bells of varying sizes, and with a loop and a stitch were ready for the weekend. When the hordes arrived in town, they slipped bells around their necks, and on wandering the packed seafront, bell-mania even drowned out the sounds of beachside donkeys.

THE DRUID IN THE GREENHOUSE

With the arrival of the modern way came a mindset to remove and stamp out the old ways of the Victorians, yet sadly in the process many fine buildings including rows of red-bricked terraced houses were demolished. Replaced with concrete structures, monstrosities of high-rise soulless places of existence, which was expertly summed up in the song 'Yellow Taxi' sang by an impish busker, below her multicoloured cap. By now, the eye of the mind was consciously opening, and with the aid of my grounding in scouting, I started the long feel of weekends by hitch-hiking to the north of the region. Meeting up with like-minded young from the cities and towns, sitting in caves and on lakeside shores before open fires, taking pleasure from the stories and songs of busking folk. Opinions and views of socialism, Vietnam and the banning of the neutron bomb were all on the menu, but although I did have a strong pull to the latter, it was mind expansion which lay at the forefront of my personal endeavour. I became inspired to seek out and purchase my first books; in fact, the only ones I could find available at the time were *Mahayana Buddhism* by Christmas Humphreys, and *An Introduction to Zen Buddhism* by D. T. Suzuki. They were soon to be followed by a short series of opportunity for its author Lobsang Rampa. *The Lord of the Rings* by JRR Tolkien, the enthralling tales of shamanic practice with *The Teachings of Don Juan* by Carlos Castaneda, also a book on Hopi Indians.

For me, on reflection the 1960s were inspirational, and I do realise that I was fortunate to live in those times, for there was a magic in the air, a Western thing that was beyond just being young, a newness that gave rise to an early realisation of potentiality. And as the windows of perception opened, a pathway to the ancient beliefs of the East, and that of all Indigenous people of the ancient places lay before me. But in a time long before the internet, there was little available in the way of gaining knowledge, never mind instruction. Local people returned from London with leaflets and magazines, and the hidden observer could have watched me attempting to meditate. And in tune with a gifted Ulster man who later laid down a collective of 'No Guru, No Method, No Teacher' I realised I was all alone with a mind full of monkeys. Driven only by a strong inner sense of destiny's path, and whether it led me to a sunken chest of fool's gold, I cared not, for it just felt right.

But as the midsummer rain fills the thirsty reservoir, I began to drink from a broadening pool of resources, I learnt more about Siddhartha Gautama Shakyamuni, the one we call the Buddha. And how the rich young prince had one day left his palace and became mortified as he observed the suffering of all beings. On taking the decision to leave his family and rich surroundings, he became an ascetic, one who is dedicated to follow a path of physical hardship, in search of nirvana.

But in time Siddhartha realised that it was not the physical hardship that would bring about illumination, but a middle way. And so, it was, after many years of practice, he sat down below a Bodhi tree, and with the conviction to remain there seated, no matter what physical or mental pain and suffering was to befall him, die or gain enlightenment was his chosen path. The rest is history for we know that he succeeded, but it was the content of learning during that experience that was passed on to us, and over two and a half thousand years later, it is still there to be read, to hear and to practise.

And so, in semi-secret and whilst lacking the modern aids that we now take for granted, I persisted with the practice, and like most newbies adapting themselves to any discipline, it did not come easy. But by allowing the toe to dip deeper into the waters of the teachings, I learnt that by consciously controlling the breath, the movement and the chattering of the monkeys began to ease, and small periods of inner peace began to unfold. I gradually obtained some knowledge of the Four Noble Truths, and the learning of two sides of the same thing, of how physical pain and suffering were connected. I had heard tell that everything was an illusion, and that time as we perceive it does not exist, but for now those secrets lay across the waters, and I did not have access to a suitable boat.

Being an only child had allowed me to slip unnoticed into the pattern of the flowered wallpaper; I often listened to the older ladies talking about suffering, even seizing bragging rights for having suffered the most. At the time I had likened their tales to the story of Jesus, as he hung nailed to a wooden cross.

But although I was not totally aware, I did see that one's lifetime on earth is not for dwelling, but for living, for we all bide in such a beautiful place, and with desire a positive mind can be trained to overcome the hardships of physical existence. And as the seventies came into being, it was John Lennon in his Gandhi-style spectacles and George Harrison with his Indian-influenced style of music that swayed my interest. For they both sang the same song, the one of love, yet from active and passive approaches: John's powerful *'Give Peace a Chance'* whilst George's gentle guitar dried its watery eyes, his mantra *'My Sweet Lord'* was delivered with a mind of abiding joy, as unconditional love flowed out to the suffering masses of Bangladesh.

Yet sadly their work was completed for this time, as they both left this physical realm at an early age. It was to be around five years after his passing, that I experienced a very vivid dream-state meeting with George.

The clarity of colour vision remains to this day, it was an experience that aspired me to go much deeper into the teachings of Lord Krishna, and in turn the Bhagavad Gita. The Gita, an epic scripture, a spiritual foundation whose teachings lay at the heart of the Hindu people.

UNIVERSAL LIFE FORCE

On the streets and out in the fields, progressive and glam rock had given way to revivalist movements, new wave, punk, and romantics.

Once again, the new generation were demanding change.

But like many before me I had entered the role of fatherhood, and with a mortgage at a time of high interest rates, the seeker within pitched up at base camp. But as a rising fish creates a circle on still water, I joined a martial arts school. A student of Wing Chun, the close combat style of Cantonese Master Ip Man, with further teachings to that of a similar style to his student, the legendary Bruce Lee, and his martial arts expression of Jeet Kune Do.

It was a Saturday lunchtime, whilst visiting a music mart, you know the one, an event with numerous stalls, huddled together inside a large soulless auditorium. Wandering the aisles in a relaxed mode of take me to where the lost sounds still play, I felt myself drawn to a particular stall. On flicking through a deep stack of vinyl, one cover caught my attention, a depiction of a colourful family of togetherness, mystical folk, gathered below a bank of trees in wintertime, an album known from times past. On purchasing, handling, and observing the album at closer quarters, the turning sparked a rekindling motion. And as black bear emerged from his winter cave, I slipped out of my spiritual torpor.

After a break in any type of discipline or relationship, and in line with the changing of the seasons, one can never return to how it once was, but with renewed vigour and a desire to achieve, I took the decision to meld my past meditation practices with that of cultivating chi.

However as with most things in life, these practices once again came with demarcations, man-made barriers, ancestral separations, ingrained by association, likes, and dislikes protected by egoic stealth.

For the chi of the Chinese, the prana of India and the Japanese ki were one of the same. Yet still at a time when practices outside the norm were laughed down or even frowned upon, the mention of Chakras, Nadis, and Yin and Yang could still be viewed as heresy in some quarters. Yet being a scholar of forward thinking, the established wheels of conditioning, simply did not fit the groove.

Growing up I recall the whispers, that he or she had turned, as mixed marriages between those that supported the Crown or Rome were still frowned upon.

During adolescence, young friends were separated and dispatched to different schools, where a lifetime of division had been intentionally created.

But below the surface and unknown to me the workings of the Dharma teachings continued to manifest. As a student

THE DRUID IN THE GREENHOUSE

of Wushu I had learnt the technique of Shaolin breathing, a method of withstanding blows by breathing with the lower abdomen. Conscious of being centred, grounded whilst either standing or seated, and with a straight back consciously allowing the muscles of the body to remain relaxed, thus enabling the breath to flow more freely. In fact, learning life-changing and life-saving techniques that really should be taught to all young children as an integral part of the Western school curriculum.

One evening whilst sharing a meal with three others, the conversation was directed towards religion, and when asked if I believed in God in Heaven, I instinctively replied that I believed in God within. Apparently, I had given the wrong answer, but although I could not expand on my statement, it had risen with a knowing from deep within, and I was happy to go with that.

Interestingly a couple of decades later on another continent whilst having a spiritual conversation with a work colleague, he simply stated that he believed in God within, and then followed that up by saying that he had no idea where that had just come from (smiley). During this period, my meditational practices had actually developed into a system more attuned with that of a fighting monk.

An increased awareness of the elements, of sensory movement, a response to a sudden change. That sharpness of being alerted to the path of a falling leaf as it made its way to earth from its tree-based Zen home, seated high in the chimney pot of a disused cotton mill.

And with it, egotism, the effect it has upon us, usually

not for the better, and how it is easier to detect in others, yet not so our own. For whilst observing ego in others, at times you can see the whole exaggerated act played out. From an early age we learn how to manipulate, the laying of bricks, to overcome hardships, to gain advantage, and the enjoyment felt from doing so. Those actions that feed the role of Me, the illusionary self, and in that process further concealing the truth. Interestingly a reverse process can sometimes be observed when an older person reaches the final stages of life, the bricks in the wall start to come down, a process that may well be illuminating for some, but sadly like the saying 'cracking up' it may bring total confusion and fear to others. Since my early years, at times, I felt a strong sense of knowing what was about to happen or may well happen in the future, with deeper feelings of premonitions, and the ability to instantly recognise different sides of an issue. As a lone and silent practitioner, I came to realise that with a strong desire to seek out certain knowledge, or to find something, then I only had to ask my inner self, the one beyond the everyday body and mind, and then to stay patient whilst consciously observing for signs of acknowledgement.

But how did I know I was asking the correct one, and not the egoic-influenced self?

SANDS OF TIME AND THE WIDENING APPROACH

The circle widened when I received a phone call, accepting an offer of employment from an American Oilfield Service company, the place of work, North Africa. And with the day of departure imminent, the hand of fate clenched its fist. News broke of an incident outside the Libyan embassy at St James's Square in London, a crowd of students had gathered to demonstrate against President Colonel Gaddafi, when shots were fired from a first-floor window. Eleven people were hit by gunfire, one of the victims being 25-year-old Metropolitan Police officer Yvonne Fletcher who was fatally wounded.

The shooting incident triggered an 11-day siege of the embassy, the deportation of 30 Libyans and the severing of diplomatic ties between London and Tripoli. It was another five months before relations resumed, when I received a sudden phone call informing me that it was time to go, it was welcome news, but there was still a feel of caution in the air.

The company had an agent in Malta, and after an evening flight I was met at arrivals and taken to a Sliema hotel, with instructions to attend the office the following morning. On arrival the agent informed me that there was a delay in obtaining my visa, and I would have to remain on the island for a further six days. On my return to the hotel, I was allocated a first-floor corner room with large window; it had excellent views of the sweeping promenade, and with a welcoming breeze all was well. After a week of acclimatising to the heat of Malta in August or so I thought, the stay ended when a driver arrived to take me to the airport for the evening flight to Tripoli.

On arrival in Tripoli and clearance of passport control, I was met by a local man with a friendly face and a broad smile; he shook my hand, directed me to his vehicle and whisked me away to the company staff house. Of course, Libya was a closed country, and on the journey from the airport I observed large numbers of marquees with outside seating, meeting places bearing green flags and material slogans about committees everywhere. The 'Green Book' the political philosophy of the Libyan leader Muammar Gaddafi came to the fore. On late arrival at a large traditional Arab flat-roof building, I was greeted by friendly staff and allocated a bunk bed in a shared room for my first night's stay in the capital. After a night of clattering air-con units, I was informed that there would be a further six-day delay, before being granted permission to travel down to the desert. Eventually clearance was granted, however, a further hold-up came when we were informed that all the desert flights were fully booked. And during the heat of the midday sun, myself and two other new Brits climbed into a car and set off on a long journey down to the company's main oilfield base camp.

On stopping for relief and in search of refreshment I went behind a closed garage building, and to my awakening, there before me on a low wall lay a row of a dozen large heads, standing erect on severed necks, some with eyes still open. I had expected to see camels on the way down, but that was pushing it. Then after a thirsty nine-hour drive and a short night's sleep, I adjusted to being driven for a further five hours south across mixed desert terrain, down to the southern oilfields of the Libyan Sahara Desert.

Although it had passed the peak of summertime, one would never have known, the days were incredibly hot and very dry, and whilst working outside on the exposed oil wells it was a physical task that I had to overcome.

The company's Landcruiser had head-height external frames fitted for 25-litre water containers, and on my first day working in immense dry heat, and much to the amusement of my two new work colleagues, I would drink a cup full of water, then spend a couple of minutes working, before rushing straight back to the water container to replenish. As a newbie one had to adapt very quickly, and on doing so learnt about desert life, its night-to-day temperature changes, sudden gusts of wind, its moods, its trickery, its brutal harshness, whilst remaining a place of beauty, with a curl of loveliness.

Winter in the desert can last for a few short weeks, and with a sudden change of cloud formation springtime can arrive, and this found me at a spot located on the edge of the Calanshio Sand Sea.

It was a mid-afternoon, whilst out in the truck on a mission with a Maltese colleague that the lads labelled Foxy, we were driving along an open sandy area in a southerly direction. The oncoming hot winds were unpleasant, and the fast-moving multi-red sky created a strange and eerie feel, an angry setting, more at home with a JMW Turner than any photograph.

Being early spring the birds from the sub-Saharan regions were beginning to migrate, and up ahead we spotted a change, a strange undistinguished commotion, on entering what felt like a curtained area, we suddenly realised that the migrating birds were in real trouble. The heat of the wind above was horrendous, and the birds were struggled to cope, they were falling out of the sky with a sudden jolt, as they hit and bounced on the hot desert surface.

We quickly pulled up and leapt out of the vehicle, emptied boxes from the rear of the truck, and began running around picking up the birds that were still alive. We had an instinctive plan to collect as many as we could and take them to a safer place. But the situation quickly deteriorated into one of horror, as hundreds were falling and landing all around us, our attempts to rescue them were futile; with full boxes, and dying finches in our hands, we realised that we had entered a realm of total helplessness. With the acceptance that life is tough, even cruel, we had no other choice but to turn our backs, climb back into the truck, and drive on in silence.

My company had its own base camps set up at strategic points around the desert, and in accordance with contractual agreements, arrangements to stay over at isolated drilling rig camps or larger sites had been implemented.

At the time, I recall it was around Ramadan, and whilst

THE DRUID IN THE GREENHOUSE

working and staying at a Libyan Oil company camp called Messla, two of us rose early, and after breakfast, set off to drive down to our company office, based inside the main camp of the Sarir Field.

About halfway through the journey I became ill, and I mean really ill, and with it the feeling that I really didn't care anymore, and all I could do was to slide down the side of the cab door and tuck myself up into a foetal-like position.

On arrival at the large camp, I managed to sit myself down on a chair inside our company office, but it became a general concern when I had to rush to the toilet to vomit, and when asked if I could make the journey back to my base camp, I had just enough energy to shake my head.

And so, a decision was taken to find a bed in the camp, a site that had chalet-type living accommodation that would not be out of place at a 1950s Butlin's holiday camp. As our company had a contract to maintain the fields Xmas trees (well heads), we were allocated rooms for rotational staff, luckily for me one was empty. I was ushered to a centrally located room with two single beds and a bathroom, the entrance door faced a pathway that led to the camps large dining room. I had stayed in the room on a previous occasion and was aware that a metal grid cover installed on the pathway clunked every time someone stood on it, and at busy times it sounded more in tune with a gong from hell than that from the start of an American movie.

But it was not the pathway that gave me trouble it was the increasing pain in my stomach and coupled with a rise and fall in body temperature I realised that I was in for a tough time. Whilst lying in bed I slipped away into a mode of high fever, only to be suddenly awakened by the churning of my insides, and as I leapt up and rushed into the small toilet, had to endure the motion of fluid passing from both ends. After a session in the loo, I staggered back to bed, and began to shiver, an action that turned into shaking, accompanied by a rhythmic drumming of uncontrolled teeth chattering, and with alternating hot and cold sweats, in a land far from home who could I turn to: 'No one' that's who.

I managed to stagger across to gather more blankets from the adjoining bed, and on throwing them down, climbed underneath the huge pile. As darkness fell, its arrival brought the sound of many strange voices, and the clunking of the metal grid transformed into teams of riveters, hammering away at a huge vessel inside a Harland & Wolf shipyard.

Sometime later I became gripped with fear, brought back into semi-awareness, as I found myself striking out, whilst under attack from gruesome beings. Distorted dinosaurs, multi-headed monsters, screeching serpents, and ferocious dragons were all trying to kill me, and with no other option I climbed out bed, drew out an imaginary sword and attacked. After a round or two I collapsed on the bed, returning to delirious sleep, only to be awoken, for the fight to be resume once more. At one-point I recall rushing to the bathroom turning on the tap, and with face submerged just drank and drank, sat down on the loo trying hard to focus, to bring reality to the fore. They came again, and at that stage I lost all reality, existing only as an otherworldly chalet fighter, a desert Don Quixote, lost in time.

After a series of battles, and whilst lying exhausted, I started to become aware that the gaps between the fighting were getting longer, and the sounds of the Belfast shipyard were becoming more distant.

I was slowly becoming aware of some normalcy when the door of the room opened and I found myself looking and talking to an Irish medic, and on taking my temperature he stated that it had come down to just under 104 degrees Fahrenheit. I discovered I had been fighting the demons for three days and nights; the medic informed me that he had been in to see me on a couple occasions, that there was a hospital on camp, but it wasn't a good place, and he really hadn't wanted to send me there.

A couple of days later I was escorted back to the Messla camp, and with the brightness and the heat of the midday sun beating down, our lonely white vehicle rose and fell in a vast sea of sand, and once again I found it hard going. On arrival back at my camp I was met by a young Libyan Petroleum Engineer, who aggressively accused me of drinking, I recall pushing past him, not even bothering to respond to his accusations. I had lost a lot of weight; my hair was matted and with a mouth and lower nose covered with blisters looked a mess. However, after a shower, a change of clothes and greetings from work colleagues and a bite to eat, I started to feel a lot better. The following day I visited the site's Egyptian doctor, a friendly chap, a philosopher with a zest for life. He confirmed that I had classic Virus1 Herpes, due to having had either sandfly fever or severe food poisoning, but it was probably the latter.

Over the coming days and weeks, it was the fighting of the demons that had played on my mind, and in summary, a realisation that they were my own inner fears, the very ones that dwelled deep down within the darkness of my being. And unbeknown to me at the time, it was something that I would confront in more detail.

At the end of a working spell in the desert we were given a field break, a leave to go home, and the journey from the desert to Tripoli was not always an easy one. Depending on your whereabouts, options of air travel were available. If you were lucky a F28 short-range jet could whisk you to the city. Or you may get a seat aboard a twin-engine turboprop F27, an aircraft that carried around 50 passengers, a flight that sometimes stopped at the coastal Sirte airfield. When a journey was made in the heat of summer, the aircraft turned around across the cooler Mediterranean Sea; it provided a physical sensation, an experience that arose from of a sudden drop of around 2,000 ft. Another option was a Twin Otter flight to Benghazi Airport, followed by a connecting civilian flight over the Gulf of Sidra to Tripoli. Or if you drew a short straw due to cancellation of flights or no available seats, then a long drive to Tripoli was the only option. After weeks of working down in the desert, whichever way you got there did not really matter, for after an evening flight to Malta, or a night in the staff house, with an international flight out the following day. Either way you would embark on a journey to another world, the one we call the West.

On the surface, the excitement of going home for a holiday remained at the forefront, but after a few years of the repetitive cycle of living in a desert environment amongst men, and then to suddenly be whisked away back to the material world, and a family home setting, can bring confusion to mind.

And eventually for me, it gave rise to a feeling of which one am I, who is me, and what is my purpose beyond the quest of the dollar? Apart from the obvious financial gains it provided the means to travel away on family holidays, and that continued to be a main driver.

During my time at home on field break, I continued with studying the Dharma, with daily meditations, and attending martial arts sessions. The marvels of hill walking had come back to the fore, with full day outings to Cumbria and North Yorkshire no matter what the weather held in store, and apart from the fitness angle, it was the oneness with nature that took me beyond the enthusiastic level. Around a week from the end of the field break, return flight tickets would arrive in the post. In fact, due to the political instability in Libya, it was the only real confirmation that you still held a job. It was just prior to the solstice of the summer of 85, when my early morning taxi arrived to take me to the airport on the first leg of the return journey back to the desert. Around mid-morning whilst allocated a window seat, the Lufthansa A737 touched down at Frankfurt Airport, and with the imaginary firing of a starting pistol, individual passengers unbuckled their seat belts, rose up and started to open the lockers, and as you know, this starts off a chain reaction. For as the aircraft taxied along the apron to its designated arrivals spot, I received a sudden strong feeling that all was not right, and on looking through my small window, a baggage truck came into view. The plane was not travelling fast, but as its port-side wing came into line it clipped the side of the baggage truck, the contact sent the aircraft into a slow spinning widdershins motion. And with a third of the passengers standing, it gave rise to a scene of chaos, people went flying down the aisles, some falling whilst helplessly grasping at the air for support. Sprawling on top of each other on the aircraft floor, screams rang out as open lockers emptied their contents of hand baggage and duty frees onto the helpless bodies below. Interestingly for the observer, the whole scene was acted out within the spinning motion of timeless movement. The aircraft eventually straightened up, the cabin crew took control, an announcement ordered everyone to return to their seats, and as we slowly made our way to a place of safe docking, a sort of normality returned.

So why did the passengers do that? Well, deep down its fear, an action to bring about a sudden closure of the airborne experience, a fear of missing a connecting flight, or simply being late, one that a seated watcher could simply call an act of impatience. In summary, that could have been me sprawled on the floor, and from a health and safety viewpoint, it was a near miss, an action that I would never repeat. On disembarking, I was not to know that the runway incident would not be the only memorable act that would come into play that day. With time on my side, I looked up at the flight departures board to discover that my connecting Libyan Arab Airlines flight to

Tripoli had been delayed. With this being a fairly common occurrence, I had options whether to leave the airport for a while, to go and eat, go to a bar or the airport shopping mall. I decided on a takeaway dish and a soft drink, to find a quiet place to have lunch, do some meditation, read a book, and just simply relax. Having casually wandered the concourse, I found a quiet spot inside an empty departure hall, chose a seat, sat back, and settled down. After a good while it started to get busier, check-in and security staff appeared, I watched as they struggled to raise an EL AL board, the flag carrier of Israel Airlines, and with the arrival of the first passengers, it was a signal for me to depart. On vacating the seat and gathering my belongings, I slowly made my way towards the Libyan Arab Airlines flight's departure lounge.

After a non-eventful flight and clearance at Tripoli Airport I was met by a friendly local driver and taken to the company's staff house, where on arrival I was informed that a terrorist attack had taken place at Frankfurt Airport, resulting in the death of three with two being young children and 74 people injured. It would be a few days later that I learnt that the incident had occurred in departure Hall B, where an explosive device had appeared to have been placed among seated passengers, with the bomb tearing a hole in the lounge floor, a second device found and defused; in fact, the very location where I had sat down on that eventful day. A number of groups claimed responsibility for the attack, whilst investigators claimed that Libyan leader Colonel Gaddafi may have played a role in the attack. How close to home, and yet so far away, was

I. After spending some time on deeper explorations, and with some trepidation I had to admit that I was receiving strong premonitions, an insight into deeper workings, I had always done so, yet since my recent life-threatening illness it had moved on to another level.

After finishing work in the desert, if we chose, we had plenty of time to be alone with our thoughts, read novels or to develop chosen practices, whether learning how to play a guitar, studying, or learning a foreign language. For me I continued with kung fu, yoga and meditation practices, along with study and gaining knowledge of the ways of diverse cultures and their belief systems. A new one I had chosen, or should I say chose me: a book on self-hypnosis. Sat alone in the room, having prepared myself, I laid down on the bed and took to the practice, it surprised me as to how quickly I succeeded.

After a brief time, I decided to lay down my intentions, and those actions bore fruit with much clearer and distinctive images, in what the North American Indians may refer to as dream time, but all I can say is that mine didn't pull its punches. During this period, the monsters stayed with me. In fact, they had remained just below the dark surface of consciousness, and I discovered that they were quite easy to access, but on doing so, I felt deep pain. And with a growing awareness that the demonic beings may have built up over this and countless other lifetimes, I took to a deeper learning of death, the afterlife, reincarnation in another material body, as the Dharmic religions and the Indigenous tribes of planet Earth believed.

FLAT TOP, THE FACING UP AND THE COMING OUT

The company's main camp was located at the foot of the Zelten Mountains, the location of the first oilfield in Libya. Whether the mountain at the rear of the camp exceeded 1000 feet I did not know. But well heads were installed on its flattish top, and in order to conduct scheduled work programmes, similar to the toy trains in India, the steep wraparound road made vehicle ascent an interesting challenge. The views from the summit were stunning, but most intriguing was the compelling atmosphere, one difficult to describe. It had a powerful all-knowing feel from long ago, a sort of 'ask me a question and I may provide you with the answer' sort of place, one where I would have liked to have spent social time or even camped out. Looking back, I now wish I had.

Over the coming nights the flat-topped mountain started to appear in my dream time, then on awakening and throughout the day I felt its pull, and on turning to view, its shape became more pronounced; on later reflection I realised it was trying to make contact, but the reason I knew not. It was a couple of weeks later and early in the morning whilst alone in a trailer

I got a sudden and very strong urge to sit down on the floor and meditate. Upon closing my eyes, I was instantly shown a clear view of the mountain, then a change as the flat top rose to form the shape of a volcano. As it grew it emanated power, and I found myself looking back from a location on the opposite side of the valley. Whilst remaining seated in yogic pose, my insides started to stir in an active motion, I observed a thin line of black smoke rising, and as it rose, a physical pain responded in tandem.

Within the increasing density of darkening smoke came loud screeching sounds, shapes began to emerge from the erupting mountain, I had no option but to reach for the waste bin. At first huge ugly horse-like beings, shrieking and writhing in sheer agony rose from the smoke-filled top, and once out, slid slowly down the front side of the mountain. Halfway down they came to a halt, remaining alive, only to be pushed further down by others arriving behind them. With the noise of sheer terror increasing, dinosaur shapes, large snake-like beings with enormous heads began to rise. It was at this point that I erupted into fits of violent vomiting; I was aware that I had returned to the chalet room in Sarir, the monsters were the same, but this time I had the advantage. Removing them from the depths of my being was not easy, as I too responded to their agony, sweating, writhing, and retching, driven on by a single-pointed desire to finish them off, I just hung on in there. Within the process a decent amount of the top layer of demons had been removed, but the remaining and more frightening ones became harder to get out. I had to work on each one individually; in

THE DRUID IN THE GREENHOUSE

fact, some only got their heads clear before sliding back down into the hidden depths. And it came to pass, I just couldn't go on any longer, although there was still plenty of work to do, I brought the session to a close, and told no one. In the days that followed the experience, I was aware of the feel of inner cleansing, a release of the deep ancestral genetic fears. I had been given a healing technique, a shamanic ritual, one that I would return to and go on to evolve and practise in later life.

The whole experience had given me a little insight into the inner battles that Jesus of Nazareth and Buddha Shakyamuni had to endure and overcome, as they faced their own demons during their quests for enlightenment, and with that in mind, field break time came around once again.

With it came the opportunity to experience new horizons, ones with spiritual connections, and after one week at home, it was back on a flight to neighbouring Egypt. For I had long been inspired by the work of Howard Carter and having previously visited a Tutankhamun exhibition, it was a visit to Karnak and the Valley of the Kings that brought about new realisations.

Arriving during the heat of summer was not ideal, but an early start provided some respite, a tang of excitement in the breeze as the little dhow made its way across the cooling waters of the Nile, towards the West Bank.

On arrival and being met by a cluster of willing guides who informed us that the tomb of King Tut was closed, and so it was the mortuary of Hatshepsut, the statues of the Colossi of Memnon that embraced the morning.

On a return visit, it was the feeling of exuberance one felt upon entering the tombs of Seti II and Ramses III, as I recall the walk down the sloping corridors, observing the painted images, some familiar but most not, but all telling the story of the way of the ancients to those in the know.

But for me it was the East Bank and the remains of the huge temple of Karnak and the energy present at the still-standing obelisk that opened my doors.

The learning of the gods of the sun and the moon, the belief of the ancient Egyptians, travelling through the underworld at night, struck the gong of most interest. For it was to Isis the wife of Osiris, the goddess of healing, magic, and the moon that inspired me to come away with new parchments of learning.

Yet it would be another decade before I physically stood before the mummies in Cairo. But it was not just Egypt that came to the fore, it was the history of the region that appeared on my radar, the Greeks, and Selene the Titan mother goddess of the moon, whilst the stories of Atlantis further stimulated my imagination. And as the juggler adds more spinning plates to his sticks, it was an act of mind management, for they all appeared so different, yet in truth were the same. Simply different paths through the forest or routes across waters that eventually come home to rest in the same place, a one that some may call nirvana. But of course there is not a place, a building with a hanging sign, where on completion, a weary traveller can claim a free pint of ale.

At times, life can be challenging on many levels. In fact, we may constantly react compulsively throughout the day, a sudden rise of anger, joy or disappointment, a statement from the media, a call from a friend, a recalled memory upon hearing a tune. The sound and sight of a red robin on a fence is a good mood indicator: does he just blend in unnoticed, remain an image on a card at Christmas, or does the bird fill you with a loving warmth, a joy to behold. Buddha Shakyamuni taught his followers to bring about the cessation of suffering by following the Noble Eightfold Path. And with words of meaning from an esteemed Tibetan Lama. 'Don't just believe in what I say. Go and find it out for yourself.'

WIRELINE MAN

Various oil companies controlled the Libyan fossil fuel fields, and with wells and installations spread across a wide area of the desert, it called upon a multi-international workforce to make it all happen. Mobile drilling derricks were installed to work over existing wells, whilst others ventured out to drill new wells in the more remote locations. A significant part of our job came towards the end of a drilling rig operation, called the completion stage. Without wishing to get too technical, the well completion comprises of running tubulars and securing downhole equipment into the lower section of the well bore. During the completion stage operation, and to stop the well bore contents from flowing up the well, it is filled with salt water and in some instances brine. To allow for testing during the completion stage, retrievable valves and plugs were inserted into the landing nipple seal bores of the downhole equipment. Our job was to rig up surface equipment, resembling a giant fishing rod and reel, loaded with 20,000 feet of wire, a means to run retrieving tools down inside the tubular to depths averaging 10,000 feet.

Sometimes and much to the delight of the rig crew, the job

went right, and like a stage act taking their final encore, the dust from the wheels of our vehicles rose in the desert air, as we sped away.

But I recall the day when two of us were called out to a rig a few hours' drive away across a varying terrain of hard compact gravel shale, dunes, and waves of soft sand. And as darkness fell with the rig site set down behind dunes, we had to look out for the sight of a light on the top of the derrick, whilst homing in, the vision of the monument of misery came into view.

Having already worked on a local well for most of the day, we lived on hope street. Maybe the company man would inform us that they would not be ready for us until dawn, and so food and beds would be made available in the nearby rig camp. But in common with the feeling of icy water lapping over the top of your wellies, the rig was ready for us to start work.

One thing we had learnt, was the ability to stay awake for exceptionally long periods at a time, and on this occasion the job went wrong.

The sun had risen and fallen a couple of times, and during the warm and windless night, we came under increasing pressure from the American oil company representative. And with no sign of a relief crew, it was one of those times when we had to draw upon our deepest inner strengths, to merely survive. Stuck out in a crazy location away from any form of normality, deprived of sleep and bordering on hopelessness, and in an altered state of mind, a strong urge of positivity rose from deep within, it was crazy, but I decided to go with it. Leaping out of the truck and with rig boot and pipe wrench, I drew a large circle in the sand, and allowing myself to go with the flow, I was carried away in a dance and chant, one akin to a North American Indian ritual. Then on ceasing all movement, I instinctively faced the south and sent out a call to the ancient powers of the land to come to our assistance. Within a short space came a reply, a signal, a feel of acceptance, the sight of a change of light formation, a distant rumbling sound, and like a creature of the deep breaking surface on a wondrous sea, an outline of a huge figure appeared. An immediate awareness that I had gone too far to pull this one back. I called out to him as our protector, and asked for his help, and on doing, was met by a felt force of a different power; our spirits lifted, and with it, an inner knowing that everything was good. I felt complete respect for the power of being, and whilst managing to remain inside the circle, raised my arms and dutifully gave thanks. From that moment, like back-seat observers, everything went right, the job was completed, the company rep and the rig crew were happy, daylight came. We even had time to drive to the rig camp for breakfast, and being mentally and physically re-energised, thoughts of sleep slipped by. All that remained was to pack the equipment away, and before that thought had time to take hold, a relief crew arrived. We handed over the task, jumped in the pickup and drove home. On the way we discussed the experience of the esoteric appearance of Wireline Man, did it actually happen? Of course, it did.

It was during the next trip that we were sent back into the hostile location, one they called Atahaddi, a place that the locals referred to as Challenge, and one that we affectionately came to call the Hat. A mystical place full of sand dunes and hidden wadis, where just gaining access into the location and finding the individual wells and drilling rig camps proved to be most challenging. In fact, the place seemed alive; it had a power of its own, a spirit that did not want you there, and so to achieve work commitments one had to overcome its hardships, and the many tricks of strong resistance. As Hat newbies your vehicles would break down, get stuck in the sand or you would simply become lost within a few hundred meters of your destination.

It was commonly stated and accepted that the rigs had drilled down into ancient burial grounds, upsetting the spirits of the ancients. And it was after losing some equipment when going over the dunes, and with a few failed attempts to locate the work site, followed by a somewhat cursed attempt to conduct the job, that I decided to contact the spirit of the Hat. So, having intuitively walked off over the dunes, found a spot near a wadi, an area that could support flora and fauna, I instinctively drew a circle and fixed an altar-like setting in the sand, and having mentally prepared myself, knelt and called upon the spirit of the place. Stating that I came in peace, and respected the land, at first a light breeze, a distinctive change of energy, an unfolding presence as an ancient power bestowed itself upon me. At such moments as this, one must instantly dismiss that instantly rising feeling of 'Oh my God' I am out of my depth, one needs to hold the line. I asked the spirit of the place for permission of access and safe passage during our operations. A warming feeling of acceptance was given, but in return, a deep knowing that I would be expected to give something back.

From then on, I began to ask the spirit of the Hat for permission and safe

passage, and it was during this process that I learnt that some individual wells, also had their own spirit. When you work every day on different oil/gas wells most jobs can be performed in line with training procedures and learnt techniques. However, the odd well may have a reputation, strange things happen, and things do not go to plan. Being in the desert allows one room for strange practices, those I am sure the nomadic peoples of the region themselves upheld. Within that same period, whilst completing a rig operation in the Hat, a likeable old American company man informed me that the rig crew were installing surface pipelines from the well head out to the nearby wadi. And after we had pulled out the downhole plug, the schedule was to rig up and run equipment called coiled tubing down into the well, and by pumping nitrogen they would lift and flow the well fluids into the wadi, the very place of sanctuary for all living things. Astonished by this planned action of total destruction, an act, beyond reason, a few of us complained bitterly, but some ignorant office-bound westerner did not care. Prior to starting the run to retrieve the down hole plug, I slipped away, communed with the spirit of the well stating my intention, I asked for the powers of the Hat to work with us. And as we were retrieving the plug, on opening a small valve above the well head, gas pressure came out, and as our tools drew nearer to the surface, the pressure on the gauge began increasing. And without my feet touching the desert floor, I arrived at the company man's office, informing

THE DRUID IN THE GREENHOUSE

him that the well had come in, the coiled tubing company were told to stand down, and the fate of the wadi was suspended.

'Tis a nice thing to work together with other powers for the greater good. Having been successful, I needed to keep my feet on the ground, for I knew that the operation had been achieved, because the spirits of the Hat had allowed it. But that confirmation increased a danger for me, for along with communicating with the powers of the desert, I was having regular premonitions, an increasing knowing of what was to become, some may call it a gift, whether a nice one or not remained to be seen. The premonitions became stronger, with clear images and sounds whether awake or asleep, whilst at home or in the desert, it made no difference. One night in the desert I was awoken in sweat from a deeply disturbing experience of a major fire inside a football stadium. A few days later during a telephone conversation from a workmate at another camp, he informed me of a major fire incident at a northern English football ground. The realisation and acceptance that serious dreams and mind pictures did actually come into being in the physical world can be quite scary. The field break came around once more, but guess what, the flights were all full, so me and a workmate from North Yorkshire decided to drive into Tripoli. In situations like this, our reliefs would fly in that night and instead of taking a desert flight the following morning would drive the vehicle back down to the desert camp. In times of trouble and especially during the course of the last five weeks, tensions between Libya and the USA had deteriorated. In fact, down to a level where a military strike was imminent. The journey had gone without incident, and it was early evening time when we heard shelling / bombing coming from offshore, most likely from the American fleet out in the Med.

About two hours out of Tripoli we were instructed to pull over as military convoys carrying mobile missile launchers passed by on the way to the city, a sure sign that we were in for an experience of some kind. It was dark when we entered the outskirts of the city and were surprised to find that the military checkpoints were all unmanned, as we pushed on towards the residential area of the staff house, the streets were empty with houses in darkness.

Then suddenly the ground shuddered, missiles began to be launched into the night sky, tracers were falling, as a USA fighter jet came in low across the rooftops. The crescendo of bombing, retaliating missiles and gun fire echoed all around, and as we arrived at our destination, we could still make out the sound of wailing coming from the neighbouring houses. The front door opened and as we ran in and up the stairs to the flat rooftop, we watched on as planes came in low overhead. Within a short time, in fact 12 minutes, the air attack ended. However, military ground forces spent most of the night firing up into the empty sky, as they did the following night, and the one after that.

On the fourth day we were both fortunate to gain a seat on the first flight out of Libya, but even that was not easy, as everyone including the military at the airport were all very edgy. A normal three-and-a-half-hour flight to Heathrow turned into seven; as air clearance through France had been suspended, we made our way through Eastern Europe and beyond, and after hours in the air found some relief when I identified the welcoming site of the Montrose Basin.

The warmth of the welcome at Heathrow scored 1 out of 10, as the aircraft stayed out on an apron for an age. On disembarking it was embarrassing as multinational passengers were met by armed police, marshalled away into an outbuilding, where further armed police attempted to treat us like prisoners.

Upon leaving departures the world media awaited, but they seemed disappointed when we informed them that the Libyans had treated us with upmost respect.

> Time to chill.
> Have a listen to 'Cello Song'
> from Nick Drake's *Five Leaves Left* album.

PIES FOR LUNCH AND THE WEATHER WAS GOOD

After a long 40 days away, I arrived home feeling somewhat displaced, but after a few more relaxing in a family setting, the warmth of Western normality began to shine through. Attending weekly classes in Tibetan Buddhism and inspired by the visit to the temple at Karnak, my spiritual viewpoints and adventures continued to widen. However, I remained aware that I was still being motivated by Eastern philosophy.

Although the island where I was born and raised had its own ancient culture and belief systems, like tasty offerings laid out on a dinner table beneath a white cotton sheet, they appeared to have been intentionally hidden from view.

In short, the wheel of the evolving effects of the 1960s continued to turn, and along with older stalwarts, younger people were learning healing practices, and with vegetarianism gaining strength, the arrival of the New Age released a new wave of optimism. As a young boy fascinated with knights, I was naturally drawn to the Arthurian legend, so upon acting on a pull in that direction, my wife and I chose to spend a few days in Glastonbury town and to visit some of the ancient sites of the region. On arrival I was met with a feeling of freshness, an energy of hidden depths. With a drift of incense likened to a holy place in India, it revealed a melting pot of religious, spiritual beliefs and esoteric practices, with new ones arising, and some not yet invented, the area was filled with an experience of awakening. It brought about a very early morning meditation session sat beside the Tor, and upon raising my eye lids, I discovered I was sat amongst rabbits, lots of them, joyfulness abounds, sitting motionless I had become a feature, as they continued their early morning activities. After a positive start to the day, we loaded the car and set off on the shortish journey to Cadbury. On arrival a walk up the energetic hill to discover a place of beauty, a mystical site where the imagination ebbs and flows to the legends of old, those colourful tales that slide uninhibited as a sword drawn from sheath. In fact, I had recently felt encouraged to purchase some dowsing rods, and this was to be my first day of practice, and I did not feel let down, as they led me away to the vibrations of the unseen. The weather was good and after a picnic lunch in the sunshine, a thank you and goodbyes, we were led back down the hill, unburdened by our untold treasures. The road to Avebury was clear, and on arrival found few folk around, and being a first-timer, I was amazed at the size of the site and what it had to offer; I came away wanting more of the same. Still in a pre-sat nav era, I scanned the road map, and set off for Stonehenge, another ancient and popular site that precedes Jesus, the Buddha and many more besides. Sites of energy and power which provide the keys to the chambers of knowledge, those realisations with that of the universe.

I had been inspired and came away with a desire to learn more about the ancient ways of Albion.

And as we are all sat down together, I will end the chapter by slipping on an appropriate song, one from the album of the same name, 'A Pagan Place' by The Waterboys.

AVALON TOWN
Holy thorn upon sleeping dragon. Abbey's tales still tell.
Crystals sparkle as bowls doeth sing, hands of healing generate heat.
Messages delivered from time beyond, prayer flags flutter below rooms for rent.
The Tower of Tarot stands tall beside silver disc.
Coloured waters rise from deep within, bather's splash, as green elemental looks on. A place of magic where seekers abound, colourful folk in fabrics gay
Climb higher and higher.

Des

QUIET BEFORE THE DESERT STORM

On my return to Libya things were not the same; a feeling of caution was in the air, and after a couple of weeks two of us took the opportunity to take a 90-minute drive to a small desert village. A settlement with a telecom's post office and with a few trading huts, it was not dissimilar to a place out west before the arrival of the railroad. During the journey I was aware of an inner feeling that something was going to happen, whether on the road, at the village or on our return I did not know. The road into the village was a little busy and as we waited at a junction to allow some military traffic to pass by, I noted that a man selling live goats and sheep was observing us, and as we continued to wait in line, he suddenly grabbed a sheep, dragged it across towards us, and with knife in hand proceeded to cut its throat. We engaged gear, the man gripping the struggling dying animal stared on with sky-blue eyes full of woe and hatred, it was a clear statement of what he would like to do to us.

If this had happened at home, such an action would have horrified us, but we both knew what the man meant, and he probably had good reason; we both reacted with a gung-ho response, one of male bravado.

On buying a few local stamps, posting a letter, and sampling a juice drink, my colleague rang his partner back home in South America.

During the return journey that inner feeling relaxed a little, which gave room for thought: could the underlying issue have been with the sheep man, for in another moment in time we could have been a target for the slaughterer, or was it to be something else?

Whilst travelling around and spending time alone I became aware of the many thoughts and visions that arose; I was aware and concerned that whenever I went to visit a place, whether at home or abroad, within a brief time after leaving, serious events occurred. It then increased with nationally broadcast and published incidents happening just before my planned arrival. In dream time I received visions of major incidents that became clearer and clearer and stayed in mind during most of the day. Disturbingly I received a desert call about a major oil rig fire in the North Sea, oddly it was the same person who had informed me three years earlier about the English football stadium fire. Some may call it a gift of prophecy but having no real desire to retreat and live in an obscure location, whilst occasionally giving out messages to those seeking answers, I realised I had a problem, one that a part of me liked. The premonitions became almost daily happenings, it was the fear of where it was going that I had to learn to overcome.

There had been little in the way of work since the American

attack, and the trip dragged along, and as days slowly turned into weeks, my turn to go home came around. Requests for flight seat bookings were generally given a few weeks prior to departure; however, due to weather conditions, flight delays and technical problems virtually anything could happen. It was a couple of days away from my desert departure when I started to get a nervous feeling, the rising of impending danger increased my awareness to that of a small creature hunting for food, during the hours of darkness in a predatory environment.

It is the uncertain unknowing of where, when and to whom something serious may happen that raises concern: will it be me, a work colleague or maybe bad news from back home? On rising the next morning with a realisation that this was my day to go home, it would normally fill one with excitement. However, a deep feeling that something was wrong lay deep rooted within.

The desert flight from this location was usually around lunchtime, a couple of pickups arrived with other joyful homeward-bound colleagues from our main camp. However, as we stood at the runway awaiting our flight that feeling of pending danger grew stronger and it came to the point where I started to question as to whether I should board, or not.

In locations like Libya with its ongoing isolation from the Western world, with economic cuts affecting supplies and a lack of new aircraft parts, an incident is a lot more likely than a holiday flight to the Alicante. In fact, only a couple of weeks earlier a Twin Otter with around 16 people onboard had struck an oil pipeline whilst attempting to land, causing maximum fatalities.

The F27 aircraft touched down and continued to swerve around like a carriage with runaway horses. It came to a stop, the doors opened, and one by one came a procession of sad and tired faces, those of men who had left their loved ones behind, who now had another period of mental and physical hardship to endure. There were nine of us booked onto the flight that day, and of course the oil company staff got the first seats whilst the remainder were shared by contractors and service company staff. Like lots of places in the world, having a friendly flight seat organiser with a liking for baksheesh gave the nod.

However, for reasons unknown the seat organiser had fallen out with our company. The shout to board went out, and as I queued at the bottom of the staircase, I wasn't sure if this was it; my end, my death on a poorly maintained aircraft, crashing down in a foreign land was right there at the front of my thoughts as I climbed the stairs. Once inside I was confronted by a sea of faces and not many seats. I managed to grab one but remained aware that the queue outside was still large. Would I get bumped off the flight with further hassles, and if so, would it save my life? I did not know the answer, but that strong feeling had not gone away. Sat on the runway with the heat inside the aircraft rising, it became obvious that the flight was overbooked and that spelt trouble, consciously looking out of the small window so as not to make eye contact. The flight organiser shouted at me and my colleagues to get off his aircraft. On disembarking, I felt a tremendous relief and once back outside in the flight waiting area, I discovered that all my company workmates had experienced the same fate. In fact, some had not even been allowed to board. I recall our number was made up of British and Maltese lads; we had a quick meeting and took the unanimous decision to drive into Tripoli. We had two three-seater Toyota pickups, so we took it in turns to travel inside the cab or sit outside with our backs tucked up against the spare wheel.

It was late afternoon when our white and blue trucks left the desert black top, taking a left-hand turn onto the main Mediterranean coast road that ran parallel with the Gulf of Sirte. Throughout the journey I still held a feeling of uncertainty; however, around three hours in, that strong feeling of danger returned. The sun was beginning to set. Two of us were seated in the open rear of the front white truck, our backs against the cab. I noticed that my Maltese companion had fallen asleep, with his head gently rocking against the spare wheel. It was a smooth journey on a pleasant evening as we sped along the coast road, with darkness in ascendancy I could just make out the dipped lights of the following blue pickup. But that feeling of fear had not gone away; in fact, it had become much stronger, I knew it was going to happen. Once again at such times it is the not knowing which action to take that increases the problem. Should I bang on the cab and tell them to stop? Should I get out, and if so, how did I know that my action would be the right one?

Darkness comes quickly in that part of the world, and with a lack of road lighting, cats' eyes or even road markings, we sped along at the same speed as we had done in full daylight. All of a sudden, and right on cue, the brakes came on, I knew this was it. We were swerving and shuddering, then a bump, it was not so bad at first, and I instantly thought we had got off lightly, until all of a sudden came a more powerful bang as the vehicle rose up in the air at an acute angle. I became instantly airborne, flying through darkness, as the vehicle noisily sped off on its side. Managing to remain conscious I put out both arms in preparation for landing, but as hands hit the ground, my left arm folded, sending my head down onto the tarmac; I rolled over and down into a roadside ditch. Lying there in darkness, conducting a mental scan of my body, it was the relief of remaining alive that came to the forefront. Having managed to scramble back up onto the road, in the distance the lights of our laid-down vehicle were still visible, the lads in the following truck slowly came to a stop. We gathered ourselves together; I was informed that a pickup truck had pulled straight out from behind the dunes. We had hit it side on, killing the driver, and as we spoke, we heard a death rattle, a realisation that they were now both dead. Unfortunately for us they were military men, with one of some standing.

I felt fortunate to come out with visible wounds, but my mate who had been asleep next to me at the time of impact had sustained a head injury and was in a semi-conscious condition, and with two Libyan army men dead my main concerns were for him and our English driver. Other vehicles arrived and a helpful English-speaking gent assisted by offering to take us away to seek treatment. As the truck slowly passed by the wreckage of the dead, the scene was set for another one of life's most memorable nights.

Having travelled for about an hour, the vehicle pulled into a military hospital, a place also utilised by local civilians, and after assistance we entered the reception area. We thanked the helpful Samaritan and waved him on his way.

The building seemed very quiet for a hospital, so we took some seats and waited. I became concerned for my Maltese mate, who was experiencing severe head pains; he continued to fall in and out of sleep. After a while four people in uniforms arrived: an Arab doctor, two African medics and a Filipino nurse. The doctor informed us it was a military hospital but they would help us as best they could, but unfortunately it was limited, as the building had no running water or drugs available. As I had the more physically obvious injuries they led me away into a surgery for inspection; the nurse removed the blood and mud and small pieces of road aggregates from my head and arm. After some squeezing, pulling, and turning the friendly Arab doctor informed me that I needed stitches above my left eye, I had no skin left on the bottom side of my right arm, and had sustained a dislocated right shoulder. Lying on the bed, I was informed it was going to be painful: my arm was pulled outwards against a large foot and then turned above my head, as my shoulder popped back into place. Held down and after another quick wipe, the stitching work on the gash above my left eye began, and with the nurse bandaging the arm it seemed like an age until they were finished.

The men left the surgery leaving the nurse to tidy up. She apologised for the lack of basic facilities, saying that she would go back to the nurses' quarters and return with a bottle of water and a vitamin pill, and true to her word she did. On such occasions it brings it home just how fortunate we are living in countries where water and medicines are taken for granted. I thanked her for her kindness but remained concerned about my mate, who unfortunately due to a lack of equipment and facilities was unable to receive any treatment.

It was around mid-afternoon when a senior nurse took me to a first-floor room, on entry it had four single beds, a squat latrine, two large windows and a pair of balcony doors that, upon opening, allowed rays of sunlight to come cascading into the flowery-like setting. It was then that the nurse reminded me once again that the building had no running water. I was then directed to sit and wait in a central seating area. After an age of waiting a man in uniform accompanied by an English-speaking civilian came to ask questions about the accident; he confirmed that both military men involved in the accident had died, and one was a senior officer from the adjoining base camp. They informed me I was safe because I wasn't the driver that killed them; our driver had been arrested and moved for his own safety. My mate was still sleeping on a chair in the hospital reception, and due to a lack of equipment and medication there was nothing they could do for him. Collectively we were not in a good place, a realisation of being somewhat helpless, totally reliant on unknown others, brings home the reality of cold steel. Due to a lack of air conditioning, it was extremely hot and sticky, I had been left to pass the time seated on a balcony chair overlooking reception.

The hospital didn't provide food, and it was down to caring

nurses who brought me some fruit from their own personal supply. I was most grateful for their kind actions. Feeling pretty naff and deprived of sleep, I had been nodding off in the chair whilst repeatedly awakening with a startled jump, as I relived the crash incident. After what seemed like an age of consciously going over the crash, the senior nurse arrived and informed that I could now go to the small wardroom for a night's sleep, words that brought pleasant music to my ears.

Following the nurse she opened the door, switched on the lights, and 'aargh' the nice airy room of just a few hours ago had completely changed into a scene of semi-terror. The bed, the cupboards and walls, curtains and ceiling were completely covered in cockroaches of various sizes, whilst an army of dung beetles were active across the floor. On informing the nurse that I would not be staying in that room, she apologised saying that because the building had no water the creatures came up the toilet and water pipes at night, but the doctor would not be happy. She led me back downstairs. I waited by a door whilst she discussed my case with another doctor. After an age two medics appeared and the one who could speak some English got my attention and escorted me to a rear ground-floor ward. On entry there were empty beds nearest the door, whilst the rear wall and central area had male patients in bed, their family members sat around on the floor cooking meals over gas flame fires. I was issued a long shirt and allocated a bed by the door, and on settling down with my back against the wall, observed the scene, once again it was like a movie set, it held a strange but not intimidating atmosphere.

The family members got on with their chores without paying me much notice, but it was not so much the actions of the humans that took my attention. The toilets were located in a corridor facing my bed, and on having a peep, due to having no water, human excrement could be seen piled up on the top and sides of the squat toilets, the bowls were overflowing with urine and traces of blood. But the icing on the cake was observing the dung beetles, who in large numbers were digging into the piles of excrement, then carrying out large balls on their backs, where lines of willing workers could be seen moving through the floors of the ward and into the adjoining corridors.

In Tibetan Buddhism the wheel of life revolves through six realms of rebirth and existence, with the three higher realms being the realms of gods and humans whilst the three lower realms are of animals, hungry ghosts, and hell beings; I saw myself as having entered into a lower and very real existence.

After an hour or so of lying on top of the bed, a couple of large male orderlies arrived and motioned me to follow them, we went back upstairs and they pointed at the small wardroom, I informed them that there was no way I would be staying in there and walked away to take a seat on the mezzanine balcony.

Then another orderly turned up, informing me in broken English that the doctor says I must go back to my room, but once again I refused.

The situation got worse when the three of them brought chairs over and started to intimidate me; they got closer and closer and just sat there staring. I reassessed my situation, I just

THE DRUID IN THE GREENHOUSE

couldn't spend the rest of the night in that room and that was it. By now I was past being tired and was half shutting down when one of them grabbed hold of me. Despite my injuries I was up in flash and removed him from my space. My action took them by surprise, I was prepared for anything, and so the watching game continued. I was in a physical mess and deprived of sleep, and as I nodded off, they came at me once again, only to retreat from my response. I knew their plan was to grab and bundle me into the room, but I had the greater need, for they were just three lads doing a job on a night shift, whilst I was prepared to stand my ground, no matter what the outcome. And so, we slipped back into the watch and wait game. It was then that the Filipino nurse turned up with an Indian doctor. He was quite firm and pointed to the room, saying that the cockroaches and beetles couldn't bite me. It was at that moment I got a brainwave. I knew that the Indian doctor would have to be a Muslim to work there, so I approached him saying that I was aware that Muslims didn't eat pork because they perceived the pig to be unclean. I then replied that Christians see cockroaches and dung beetle equally unclean. He instantly changed, understood my point, and informed me I could stay on the balcony until daylight, but then I would have to go into the room or I would get him into serious trouble. The nurse informed me that all the insects would be gone by then, so with my head resting on the balcony wall, I fell asleep.

Sometime later I was awakened by the nurse who said that I had to move quickly. Feeling a bit apprehensive I rose and followed her. As she entered and opened the curtains, all was well. In fact, the room had transformed into a peaceful setting. The nurse informed me that a senior doctor will be coming to see me, there was a military-style pyjama robe to wear, and I must remain in bed. Unable to wash, I was in a sweaty mess. However, I just went with the flow and fell asleep on top of the bed. I was slowly brought around by the sounds of voices, and opening my eyes discovered a crowd of about ten people stood around the bed. The head doctor was doing his rounds with students and had left me until last. Everyone was positive and friendly, and after an examination he informed me that he would arrange for me to go to a hospital in Tripoli. I told him a little untruth, in that I had a ticket for a flight to Malta that evening, and on arrival my company would get me into a private hospital. He accepted that, shook my hand and they all left the room. It must have been around midday when I was standing out on the small balcony simply staring, when a familiar pickup entered the car park. My work colleagues had discovered our location, and on collecting the two of us, I said goodbye to the hospital staff and we headed off to Tripoli.

On the way I discovered that my workmate the English driver had been arrested and would spend some time in a Libyan prison, whilst the one with the head injury had appeared to come out of the crash a lot worse than I did.

For me the immediate situation came to an end when I attended a clinic in Tripoli that evening, and on the following day took a flight home.

The knowing that I took from the experience was one of vulnerability, a realisation that we are simply a light bulb, shining bright, getting dimmer or turned off by the flick of a switch.

ONE STARRY NIGHT OUT

At a time when the embargo placed on Libya had started to bite, and with exploration and production in decline, I bizarrely found myself living alone in a trailer at a company camp located on the outside perimeter of an oil field site, named 103A.

After a long 38 days in the field the day to go home came around.

Due to a loss of revenue, our company had decided to make savings on travel arrangements, and after a cheap room stopover in Malta, four of us took an early morning Pan Am flight to London. Whilst at home that evening news broke of the Lockerbie air disaster. Yet it would be some time before we discovered that the explosive device had been placed amongst the baggage of our Air Malta flight from Tripoli, and with four of us on the Pam Am flight to London on the same morning of the bombing, it did not leave much to the imagination.

All alone in the camp I had a four-wheel drive pickup at my disposal, and with a list of clients to visit, the days were taken care of. But with spare time in the late afternoons and the midweek evenings, practices and projects needed to be implemented.

It was on one such evening I took the decision to do something that I had been planning for a while, but driving out alone into the desert at night without informing anyone of my destination was not the safest of things to do, but it certainly added spice to the experience. Like most nights in the Sahara Desert, after the temperature of the day had cooled, it lacked high humidity, which made it much easier to move around, and with the bonus of a clear evening sky I set off in a south-westerly direction.

My aim was to find a lonely spot, one free from the borrowed light of gas flares campsite lighting, and without noise. This area of the Sahara was mainly flat, made up of shale and broken shells from a one-time ancient seabed. After about a 30-minute drive, darkness was descending, and on having overcome a rising fearful sense of what ifs, I stopped the engine and jumped out of the truck.

On surveying the scene, dim lights were visible away to the east and the northern horizons, I climbed back into the truck and drove on.

At that time in evolution Sony Walkman cassette players were in vogue, and on becoming immersed in solitude and sound, I drove much further than I had intended. Returning to consciousness and guided by a strong feeling to bear to the right, apart from the movement of the vehicle's two dim headlights it was completely dark. I stopped the truck, switched off the engine and stepped out into the night. My plan was to move away from the cooling sounds of the truck's engine and into the darkness, and after a few minutes' walk whilst consciously only looking down I received a feeling of inner warmth, a sign I was there, my allocated spot. I sat down and after alignment, time spent on breathing preparation, no external sound could be heard, and with a total lack of breeze I slipped beyond the senses and into a mode of meditative awareness. After a timeless period of absorption wrapped in a parcel of peace, I slowly opened my eyes. Behold the sight of an indescribable vision of vastness, a rhythmic dance, above and all around. But it was not just the sensory vision of the night sky, it was the feeling of being alone and exposed to the powers and forces way beyond my state of being. The awareness of being a tiny energy particle of universal existence, a humbling beyond humbleness. In fact, I had to overcome a sudden rise of feeling totally inferior, and the inevitable arrival of fear. As I worked with the placement of being an unseparated part of the whole, the cosmos invited me to join in. I stood up swaying slowly at first, then glided into a movement of stepping and turning in a motion of oneness with the power of the great wheel, and on doing I slipped away into the oceans of creation.

Sometime time later I became aware of my physical self once more, and having transcended little me, I moved back to the vehicle, climbed up onto the back of the pickup, connected the Walkman, lay down on my back and watched the great free show of the starry heavens. After a feeling that my time was up, I rose and climbed back down, entered the cab, turned the ignition key, changed direction, and headed back to a place of human occupation.

It was a strange journey, one with a feeling that time and

THE DRUID IN THE GREENHOUSE

space had gelled into one, yet it was not too long before I saw the orange flares, and with it, a feeling of 'Oh well' as semi-normality and separateness crept back in.

On arrival at camp, I parked up the truck, entered the trailer, made a hot drink, opened the door, and sat down on the top step, and whilst staring skywards slipped into contemplation, peacefulness with the arrival of dawn.

The time had come for me to leave Libya before she took me.

It had certainly been an experience, and one that provided the means to form friendships. And if any of those people get to read this book, then all I can say is 'Thank you' and I send out my love to you and your families.

Om Shanti

THE SUSHUMNA EXPERIENCE

Although I had left Libya, those happenings still continued.

It was a Thursday afternoon, and after a long drive north, I booked into an Aberdeen hotel. The next day I rose feeling edgy, once again something was not quite right, and on arrival at the airport, I checked in for a fixed-wing flight to the Shetlands. During the flight I felt uncomfortable, a feeling that something was going to happen. I recall getting into conversation with the guy seated next to me, but as we came in on the final approach my thoughts were elsewhere.

A minute later as the plane touched down, the left-side wheel collapsed, the aircraft went down on the low side, and at speed swerved, and left the runway, ploughed across an adjoining field, before coming to a stop near a flock of surprised sheep. My immediate thoughts were that we had got off lightly; everyone onboard remained seated, the doors opened and we systematically climbed down on to a field of wet grass. Once we had all disembarked and got ourselves together, I realised that the uncomfortable feeling had gone away.

Whilst offshore and off-shift, when all alone in my allocated cabin, I continued with yogic practices. I was aware that when you refer to yoga, people assume it is just a physical practice. It remains a strange thing that we are encouraged to train and get ourselves physically fit, a goal that involves various forms of rigorous exercise, and yet those that also practice inner fitness may be seen as a bit odd.

In stormy weather the seagulls around the rig structure tended to group together on the same girder, so too, certain individuals would approach me with a desire to learn about meditation, and as they were obviously interested, I willingly accepted their request. But inner work has powers of its own and having introduced them to I Ching and further practices, they instinctively followed their own paths. Yet it still came as a surprise when one day I overheard an enthusiastic conversation about yogic breathing practises from two lads I did not even know. At times in life and especially after a tragic incident, people may question how such a terrible thing could have happened, and you may well have heard the phrase that 'God works in mysterious ways. Not to mention pre-birth arrangements, the natural universal law of cause and effect operates without judgement.

As we enter a new life with our pasts accumulated karma, we have free will and with it the choice to make decisions. Karma is a part of everything, yet we in the west mistakenly see it as a stick for punishment.

During a period of employment in the North Sea's central field, I had been working on a personal project, something of a far greater source and power. But trying to prove the unseen can be tricky, and during my stints offshore, when alone I continued with my esoteric practices. Having just completed a ten-day operation, I was scheduled to fly off the rig the following morning and with a couple of hours free I ventured into the TV lounge. Whilst watching and listening to a person being interviewed on the 24-hour news channel, I suddenly realised that points being raised in conversation bore a similarity to those of my own esoteric project. Then suddenly and unexpectedly my life changed, I had a profound realisation, that was it, for I had just succeeded in discovering the answer to the meaning of the universe, of infinity. When instantly a force of power shot up my central nervous system and out through the top of my head. I was completely blown away, mesmerised, and in a state of extreme bewilderment. Darkness on the left side of my brain and stars of the universe on the right, and with it a strange, distorted feeling of euphoria. I thought that I was about to die, awaiting a being from another realm to come forth and escort me away. And within the semi-darkness of the room, I just sat their staring in readiness. After a minute or so in silence I gained some sort of a grip, I was aware that something had just shot out of the top of my head. Raising my right hand with a degree of fear, I slowly slid my fingers carefully across the top of my skull, and on lowering my palm I was pleasantly surprised to find it clear of wet blood. Sat in semi-darkness in a small room with around 15 others watching television, all unaware of my situation, I remained seated, trying to fathom out what had happened, all memory of what I had been working on had disappeared, and to this day I have no recollection.

THE DRUID IN THE GREENHOUSE

However, the experience had left its mark, everything seemed slightly different, the room, people's faces, and sounds were all off key.

Upon rising I slowly made my way out of the television lounge, whilst hoping no one would speak; I managed to open the door and step outside, and whilst holding onto the handrails slowly made my way back to the cabin.

I spent the remaining time on the rig in a sort of a strangely strange, but oddly, normal mode of perception.

The next morning arrived with a chopper flight back to Aberdeen, and with a following flight to Manchester and a taxi ride home, I managed to hold myself together. Fortunately, it was Christmastime, and with a couple of weeks off, I believed I had enough time to recover, but I couldn't have been more wrong. For at home, I realised that there were sides to my condition that revealed a warped state of shock, with an increasing feeling of ecstasy and bliss. But who could I turn to for help? Can you imagine what a GP would say, or on referral what would a specialist think when I told them my story. But after a few more days rest I realised that I had a serious problem. I did confide with a long-time friend, and during a walk by the river, stopping on a bridge, the views over the water and bankside were very different to that of the norm. The whole structure of the bridge had changed, streams of silver light descended and danced along the high bank, as eyes looked on, conscious trees in movement, unison of water and air energy flowing around them and me, the effect of the experience intensified each day. As the seasonal festivities continued, I sort of got a grip, and having a stranger sense of humour anyway, to a degree I managed to get away with it.

On returning offshore, I lived in hope that it would just fade away, but everything appeared unreal, an illusion of fun, a viewpoint that most others offshore did not share. During my time alone in the cabin, I took to studying at a level of intellect way beyond my previous understanding, and with increasing spiritual realisations, I was becoming what some would describe as mad. For I knew what the time on the clock said without looking, the name of the person who was about to knock on the door, and whilst attending a meeting knew what people were about to say before they spoke.

I was conscious that some of my work colleagues were aware of the change within me, and it became more than concerning when I realised, I was in a state of a process of fragmentation, for the spaces between everyday normality and otherism were widening. Once again, I considered visiting my GP, but can you imagine telling him that one afternoon I was sat in a TV lounge in the middle of the North Sea when my head exploded, and since then I can see fairy folk, and know what's going to happen before it actually does. Although it may have been fun to watch the GP's reaction, they may well have been looking at sectioning me, and with a strong feeling that wouldn't have been the best thing for me, I stayed away.

So, in order to survive in the here and now, I had to adjust my behaviour, and like an actor learning a new role, I developed a strategy with cloaking techniques and stage presence. For I knew that the answer to my problem lay in discovering the knowledge of what had happened, and so in the pursuit of that truth, I became the seeker of my own sanity.

In order to handle the day-to-day periods, I threw myself back into my trusted physical pursuits of hill walking, Wu Shu, yogic meditation, attending Dharma classes, and with the further studying of the Bhagavad Gita, kept my head down as best I could. And as the salmon of wisdom returns to its place of birth, only to find that much on the way had changed, my journey across the sea of insaneness also provided insight and knowledge.

It was still a good while before dawn, lying there perfectly still, yet wide awake, conscious of the activities of the third eye, that initial realisation that I wasn't the body nor the mind, yet I needed confirmation. Then an eerie sound came from a pair of local barn owls, calling out to one another as they haunted the night.

But once again my Achilles heel, an awareness, for when on my travels to a location, it could be anywhere in the world, just prior to my arrival, whilst being there or having just left, something alarming may happen.

Whether driving a vehicle, having a shower, standing at a shop checkout, an image of an event would be shown to me; it could be a major blaze at a castle, a line of dead bodies in a field, a terrorist attack, tsunamis, landslides, breaking dam walls, and worst of all abductions, suicides, and murders closer to home. There was no respite, for even in dream time being an emotional observer in attendance at such events, and on awakening that feeling of being disturbed by those actions was bad enough. But it was the confirmation on hearing or watching the events being played out on national news programmes that I had to deal with. Like many before me when their lives become difficult, they seek refuge in peaceful practice. So, I dropped those physical and social pursuits, simply tuning into my inner self to seek sanctuary, and whilst guided from within, took time to explore the deeper levels of subtle practice, those of the North American Indians, and that of the Great Universal Spirit.

And amongst the swirl of a maddening mind, I found solace, and with a degree of determination I glided on, to be rewarded with realisations and an experiential knowledge in the workings of mind.

'But where is the mind? asked the Welsh lady, as she sat beside her spinning wheel, 'The mind is not of the body, but a temporary expression of pure consciousness,' replied the weaver of the yogic cloth.

With that in mind and with a few weeks of free time available, my wife and I boarded a flight to Goa. On arrival we found a cosy place to stay in Anjuna, hired a scooter, attended Dharma courses, and simply chilled out by the Indian Ocean. It was the early mornings and evenings that brought most benefit, and especially the latter, just sitting, watching, and absorbing the power of remarkable sunsets. After a period of semi-bliss, we returned to the airport and boarded an Indian Airlines flight to Bangaluru. After an interesting time, looking down onto the spine of Southern India, which is the Western Ghats, we descended into the state of Karnataka. The city of Bangaluru was clean and buzzy, with parks and distinct buildings, a place in the process of becoming the super hi-tech city that it is today.

But during our short stay a clash of worlds came about, when a large crowd of Hindu men took it upon themselves to demonstrate against the ways of Westernisation, by burning down a recently opened American fast-food outlet, and along with the arrival of MTV, I suppose it was all a fast step too far.

The following morning, we boarded the Shatabdi Express to Mysuru, and after a comfortable three-hour journey in an air-conditioned carriage, we arrived in the Sandalwood City, a delightful place, where one wouldn't have enough room on a postcard to explain its delights. The station held an interest for me, for although it was far too hot to wear an anorak, right there on a track at the rear of the station. I was fascinated to take in the sights of a couple of Swindon-built steam-powered locomotives. After negotiations with a local rickshaw driver, we arrived at our chosen destination and were fortunate to find a room in the Parklane Hotel, a city centre hangout, most noted for its courtyard bar and restaurant, and a good place to spend a week of one's life.

Whilst in the city we had to get used to airborne dust/sand particles, that at times blocked the nose and reddened the eyes. And when out and about, colourful scarfs could be seen wrapped around western faces.

Mysuru certainly has its attractions, the distinctive smell of sandalwood that drifts from its many incense factories laid down a base, whilst the smell of raw bananas ripening inside the central market's ovens, melded with that of the distinctive colours of Mother India. Overlooking Mysuru stands the summit of Chamundi Hill with its Hindu temple, a huge image of Nandi, the humped seated bull. Nandi, the mount of Lord Shiva, who along with Brahma and Vishnu form the Hindu Trinity. Lord Shiva the main Deity of Hinduism whose role is to destroy the universe in order for it to be recreated. Accessed by road, or by foot up a 1,000 steps to its 3,000-feet summit that is considered a rite of passage for visiting pilgrims. After a rickshaw journey we climbed out at the base of the hill, it was during the heat of the late morning when we started the long ascent up the stairway. Although hard going, it was inspiring to meet the very old and those we would call disabled, devoted pilgrims who with every step uttered mantras, a sacred sound that echoes through timeless existence.

On arrival at the summit, we poured bottled water over steaming necks as the rays of the sun penetrated our being. We sought a place of sanctuary, a cool drink, and a light lunch. After a time spent wandering the bazaars and hilltop sights, towards late afternoon we had to embrace ourselves in a swaying rugby scrum, in order to gain a tight standing spot, on a local bus. A bumpy journey where everyone on board including the driver wished to befriend us, it ended too quickly.

After a cool shower and a change of loose clothing, we dined out at an open rooftop terrace restaurant, a place known for delicious food, and along with a cold drink, brought an end to a memorable day Mysuru Palace is out there on its own, the seat of the kingdom, a truly magnificent structure, a gem that we actually visited three times. During the second

THE DRUID IN THE GREENHOUSE

daytime visit, with the sun high in the sky, we wandered the grounds, there were few folk about, until we came across an interesting gent and a young boy taking a drink in a shady spot. Upon striking up conversion we discovered they were of a priestly caste, and with the inspiring priest no doubt seeing the opportunity to make a rupee or two asked if we would like to get married. We informed him we were already married Western-style. He placed his hand upon his heart, looked straight into our eyes, and stated that this would be something different. After a casting glance we accepted, and he pointed to a distant structure and told us to return there in 30 minutes' time. They departed and we strolled on past the ancient steps that led down to a small shine. A little further on a sign pointed the way to a small café; we took refreshment and pondered over what we had just agreed. On time we left the café, and ahead stood the young boy in waiting; he appeared different. He requested we take off our shoes, wash our feet, hands, and faces with water sprinkled from a plastic bottle; he placed scarfs around our shoulders, and in my wife's case loosely over her head, and we followed him down the stone steps.

Reaching the bottom, we were immediately taken back by the sight before us: behold a powerful shrine full of shimmering candles, incense and flowers, images of deities, and to the right stood the priest dressed in immaculate white; he was smiling with a level of holiness that neither of us had ever previously experienced. Garlands of marigolds were placed over our heads, strips of silk ribbons and meaningful cottons were tied around our wrists, holy water was sprinkled up on us, and as mantra began, red Bindi spots were placed on our foreheads. The ceremony commenced in local tongue, tiny bells echoed as we drifted away within in its pure essence, occasionally the boy whispered detail in English, and when the moment came for the puja offering of light, our hands joined, and with the holy man's hands laid over, the power of the invoked had a deep effect upon us. As it slowly came around to a peaceful ending, we were allowed plenty of time to adjust, and after paying our respects and a modest sum, we followed the young boy up the damp stone steps. Stepping out into the dazzling sunlight, and whilst embraced with a feeling of the reborn, we walked on with a divine togetherness, a tiny vessel becalmed on an ocean of joyful bliss.

The next day our last in Mysuru, brought the big weekly event, the Sunday illumination, the evening when the palace is lit up with nearly 100,000 electric bulbs. And on leaving the hotel and joining the throng who came from near and far, the site of the huge building stood out as a distant attraction. But as we drew closer behold a fairy-tale setting, a magnitude seldom seen opened before us, and on reaching the palace we became immersed in a generated vibration of excitement. And as the hour on the clock turned to signal the end of the free show, we turned away, and with the darkened shape of the building now behind us, made our way back into town. After a last night and a full breakfast, we settled our bill, took a rickshaw back to the rail station, and four hours later, a taxi ride to the airport, where we boarded a return flight to Goa. But there was a twist, for after 20 minutes in the air we were buzzed by jet fighters from the Indian Air Force; the captain informed us that we

THE DRUID IN THE GREENHOUSE

would have to return to Bangaluru. Back inside the airport we were told that due to military operations the flight will be further delayed. One hour later an announcement informed us to re-board the aircraft, and after an uneventful flight we arrived back in Goa.

The final week saw us back on the scooter, a form of transport I had once embraced as a teenager, but the UK was often wet whereas in Goa you had to remain conscious of the power of the sun's rays on your legs and neck.

After visiting the sites, the markets, and beaches, and after numerous samples of spicy vegetable dishes, papaya, mango, and coconut juices, the time came around to hand back the scooter. Taking a last smile at a place of natural beauty, we boarded a flight and headed back home, and all seemed well in the universe once more.

The trip away had come at the right time and had helped enormously; the intensiveness of my visions had reduced to a more manageable level, and as I boarded a chopper flight back out to a rig, I felt more in control of my being. After completing the ten-day work operation, I was told I could go home the following day and being the only one from my rig going in, the admin man found me a seat on an afternoon drilling rig crew change flight.

However, on rising the next morning, that dreadful feeling had returned, the very one that something bad was going to happen.

During the early afternoon that feeling of impending danger had increased, assuming that it had to be the chopper flight that was causing concern. Should I stay or should I go now? came to the forefront. A conundrum, for if I requested, I may have been able to stay for another night, but then an incident on the rig may occur, and with the confirmation of not knowing, all I could do was link palms with the hand of fate. Being the only passenger awaiting the arrival of the flight, the rig's gas flare went out. And with escaping gas a danger to an arriving aircraft, the chopper was not permitted to land, and so I watched on, and as the supervisor attempted to reignite the gas flare with the aid of a single shot flare gun, the chopper circled the platform in the distance. But after three attempts to reignite, the flare remained unlit, and from my location in the admin doorway, I could hear the pilot on the radio requesting an update, stating he couldn't wait much longer, and would shortly abort the landing and head on into Aberdeen.

That feeling of danger had not gone away, but either way the flare had to be relit, and on the final attempt before the chopper left the area a good shot reignited the gas.

The S61 model can carry up to 30 passengers, and offshore workers have to undergo regular training in underwater helicopter escape. And it was taken as a known that there was one seat at the back of the aircraft that in an emergency ditch situation, the seated individual would not be able to get out. And as I climbed the steps to be met by a sea of staring faces, those ones who had just completed two weeks away from their loved ones, who had willingly put their life pastimes on hold, in part saw me as the culprit who was delaying their homecoming. Understanding their feelings, I made my way down the single aisle only to discover that the only remaining seat was the one, but I had known that all along. As the chopper rose up and flew away the feeling of danger had actually increased, and with up to a three-hour flight time back to the mainland, those usual nice thoughts about going home were left stored away in the bottom of my bag.

About 20 minutes out, and with an increasing feeling of anguish, the communication bell rang, an announcement from the pilot, by now I half expected him to say we were going down to ditch on the sea, but instead he stated we had an instrument reading problem and would have to return back to my rig. At that point my personal feelings of danger had spread to the other passengers, but after twenty more minutes we arrived back on the helideck, and having disembarked we all went to the mess room whilst the crew inspected the craft. After a break we were called for take-off, and once back in the air that feeling of danger had gone away. The scary bit being, like the roll of a dice on a roulette wheel, it was down to a choice, much like a badger attempting to cross a dark road at night. I had a feeling of being exposed in a game of chance, and with that in mind, I felt more relaxed. Warming thoughts of going home, meeting my family and friends, immersing myself in nature came into play.

During this period, I went on regular walks in the hills of the Lake District, North Yorkshire and my local Bowland Fells with family and friends.

And out night fishing on a low water mark with the moon in attendance, absorbing the natural energies of nature which replenishes our reason for being. Continuing with my ever-growing spiritual practices, I was consciously aware of having developed an aversion to the feeling of being proud and that of pride in general. And along with the equally important fact that I had a problem with a coincidence, it was the realisation that the Dharma and mind-training practices had been chipping away in the mode of stealth.

For when a person takes on the challenge to consciously improve their inner self, it has similarities to my experiences of hill walking, for it can actually be the start point that is usually the most difficult to find.

From my start-up days when there was next to nothing available at all in the West, it appears to have moved to the other extreme. For the arrival and growth of the New Age scene provided the seeker with a wealth of choices, organisations, numerous outlets, retreats, with individuals offering readings, healings, and techniques for awakening. And like steam rising from a bowl of hot broth, the correct path up the mountain may well appear to be shrouded in a spiritual mist, especially for those wearing glasses.

And to close on that point, how about listening to 'A Forest' by The Cure.

THE LITTLE BOOK OF AWAKENING.

The Islamic call to prayer, delivered five times each day, brings great benefit. By accepting a permanent role on a specified rig, a single room increased my capacity to study and provided the means to meditate at leisure, and starting with a 5 am session each morning, was right up my path, so to speak!

On transferring from an onshore location to the UK waters, I remained aware of the esoteric skills I had discovered and developed during my time in the Libyan desert. For there had been a number of occasions when the secret practice had brought success, and a standout one came towards the end of my stint in the North Sea. There was a particular well on a gas platform that had tools lost down a hole, and over the course of time, around five years, numerous unsuccessful attempts had been made to retrieve them. A management decision had been taken to give it one last attempt before the drilling rig moved over the well, and that remained an expensive option. We had been given a couple of days to retrieve the lost tools but all attempts had failed. On the final day with the crew gone for lunch, I took the opportunity to go down to the lower well head deck, and after preparation placed my open hands upon the Christmas tree and called upon the spirit of the well to confirm its presence. And behold, 'May peace be upon you'; I got an immediate reaction. I introduced myself stating aloud that I had come with good intention, requesting assistance in removing the alien materials from deep within.

On closing the act of invocation, I returned to the upper floor and proceeded to run the retrieving tools down into the well, it took over half an hour or so to reach the top of the lost tools, and with immediate effect latched on. Then with a slight jarring action the lost tools came free, the cab instruments showed a substantial increase in weight, and being the last day of the trip, it delivered extra cause for celebration.

After spending a long weekend at a music festival, and with the jingling bells of the folk of the Morris still plucking my strings, I felt fortunate to have the opportunity to go and experience the eastern Himalayan state of Himachal Pradesh.

On arrival at Delhi Airport, we collected our rucksacks and made our way out, whilst consciously coming to terms with the sticky smell of the early morning air. With time to spare we slowly made our way along a line of parked buses, intending to go to the domestic airport, we boarded and took seats at the rear of a Delhi bound bus. It was still dark. Throughout this time, I had observed local males moving around in a menacing manner; they were targeting young men who had come off our flight from the Gulf. Those souls who had been working away from their homes for lengthy periods, and on arrival back in India with newly acquired electrical goods and no doubt

THE DRUID IN THE GREENHOUSE

cash, were an easy target for organised predators. Young Gulf workers arrived and sat together at the front of our bus and in a short time, like scavenging hyenas, local hustlers gathered, three men jumped on board, whilst one remained on watch outside. They started to abuse the young workers, and with menacing threats demanded they handed over their wares and empty their pockets, basically they were being mugged. Being a son of Robin Hood, I couldn't turn a blind eye, I stood up and took a walk down the aisle, and whilst taking a position in the doorway blocked off the muggers exit, whilst the one outside slid away. Upon making them aware of my presence, the remaining three muggers got edgy, the workers grew in confidence, to the point where tables turned, and we could have mugged them. And with a few chosen words they reluctantly stepped off the bus. In a flash the driver appeared and off they scarpered. With a turn of a key the engine shuddered and away we went, the open windows invited the cool morning air to stream into the bouncing vehicle, the working young men came down the aisle to thank me. On reflection life can be hard, imagine working away from home for a year or so, and on arrival, having your bounty taken off you by fellow countrymen. And then on the other side of the same street, imagine you were a member of a team, who each night like a large a cat observing deer at a waterhole, waited at arrivals selecting your prey. After a short bus journey, we arrived at the domestic airport, and with goodbyes all round took our leave and checked in for the Jagson Airline flight to Shimla. On hearing the call to board, we made our way to an aircraft that back in the desert we called a shoe box, and with cargo loaded and five passengers seated, it was chocks away, and with the propeller turned by an eager attendant, the engine fired, and we were off. The plane climbed noisily to cruising height then levelled off, the weather and visibility was good, and the final approaches were interesting as a mountain side came into close contact on the starboard side. We were told to prepare for landing, but strangely it never descended, for the wheels suddenly began bumping along the top of the tabletop mountain runway. Upon climbing into an Ambassador taxi, the driver informed us we were fortunate to land, as the runway was situated at just over 1500 meters above sea level and due to severe weather, it regularly turned back. A couple of days spent at the old British summer capital of India, sampling the delights of Shimla with its Yorkshire-like high street. Our choice of hotel was down on the cart road, the night-time view from our bedroom window displayed the towns impressive church as a giant Christmas tree, a fae setting that added more fruit to the bowl of a joyful stay.

After two-nights and a breakfast we agreed a price with a local driver, checked out and set off in a northerly direction through the exquisite Kangra Valley.

A couple of hours later we stopped for chai at a small riverside café, stretched our legs, then sat absorbing the beauty, as floral scent stimulated our senses.

On completing the journey, we thanked our driver and climbed out onto a busy market street, and after a quick lunch and a look round the stalls, gained some local information about our destination. Upper Dharamshala or McLeod Ganja,

THE DRUID IN THE GREENHOUSE

sited on top of a high ridge, with two routes of access available, one straight up by foot or shared jeep taxi, or by bus along a winding road. We decided on the latter, the 30-minute journey up the mountain is quite superb, with a point of interest being the church of St John in the Wilderness with its inviting graveyard, a must-place to visit during our ten-day stay.

The bus stand of Little Tibet is located on a crossroad at the top of the ridge, and at over 2,000 metres above sea level provides panoramic views of the western plains, and the rear ice wall, which is the Dhauladhar range.

The character and atmosphere of the place is uniquely refreshing, with traditionally dressed Tibetan folk and robed monks of all ages going about their chores as though still in Lhasa, their forever spiritual home.

The place is a treasure trove for the Western traveller, with prayer wheels and flags, numerous stalls and shops selling colourful clothing and spiritual artefacts, and along with good cheap food and plenty of accommodation options, it provides ample opportunities for an unforgettable stay. Being in India for only a few weeks our budget provided opportunities to release the purse springs ,and so after a three-night stay in a basic room we chose to relocate to Glenmore.

Nestled in a wooded setting a good twenty-minute walk from town, we opted for a one-bedroomed Tibetan-style cottage. It provided a memorable weeklong stay, with breakfast and optional evening meals provided by the owner Mr Singh in his colonial type house. A splendid property that overlooked a lawned garden embraced with local flora, the song of birds and the smell of cedar wood, not to mention his dog and the visiting family of Tibetan ass. And it was here that the tranquillity and serenity of simply being, complemented the tasteful smell of flowering jasmine.

We spent our days simply chilling out, wandering around the area visiting monasteries, cultural centres whilst purchasing Tibetan handcrafts and sampling tasty food. A memorable experience being an evening trek around a hillside to attend a performance by the Tibetan Institute of Performing Arts. One afternoon we decided to walk down to the main temple, and after surprisingly going through security we sat and soaked up the atmosphere as the Dalai Lama delivered a discourse to his adoring kinfolk. Towards the end there was a break where traditional baked breads and gallons of butter tea were handed out and being a pair of only ten Western folk in attendance, the locals ensured we had more than our fill. Yet warm Yak butter tea would not be a first choice at Bettys Tea Rooms in Harrogate.

Our final night in McLeod Ganj just happened to be on the eve of Diwali, the Hindu festival that symbolises the victory of light over darkness, good over evil, knowledge over ignorance.

Mr Singh invited us to the main house for an evening meal celebration, and on arrival were introduced to members of the Tibetan Government in exile.

Prominent officials and along with another Western man brought together a collection of individuals, which gave rise to interesting conversations.

But unfortunately, due to our scheduled early morning

departure time, we had to take leave much earlier than we would have wished.

Alas we shook hands and hugged our new friends, gave our thanks for their superb hospitality and after saying our farewells to Mr Singh, it was a wrench to leave. Knowing that all good or bad things must end, we stepped out into the darkness, and made our way back to the lodge by torchlight.

During our stay at Glenmore the individual Tibetan-style lodges were in their infancy, and during our visit we held discussions with Mr Singh about the prospects of future development, and the market strategy for his business.

It was a few years later we learnt that world-famous celebs including Richard Gere, Paul Simon, and Martin Scorsese were amongst the guests that have since stayed at Glenmore.

It was still dark when the young driver arrived, and after loading our packs we set off on a journey down to the plains of the Punjab, to board the Pathankot Express train to New Delhi. As the journey progressed the first rays of dawn played an intro to the awakening of a new day, magnificent flora and fauna in the Himalayan foothills, a journey for the sheer pleasure of living.

An hour and a bit later we pulled up at a hilly roadside stall, our senses were alerted to the warming smell of cardamom drifting out from a balanced lid above a large urn of sweet chai, and with a sticky bun in attendance, provided an ample start for the long day ahead. But it was the feel of the energy of place that really caught my attention, for within a short walk from the food stall the prana of the morning hung tastefully heavy, and within the mystical rising mists, our humming hearts shared blessings with the birth of a brand-new day. In India and in yogic practices they call it prana, within the dojos of martial arts qi or ki, the energy of Reiki, whilst in movement at the banks of rivers, chi. Whereas a Celtic Druid may consciously refer to the magical energy of Nywfre.

Whether universal life force or the pure essence of gods breath, a name is a word spoken, for the happenings just after dawn can be simply sublime, and in the knowing that all is well in the world, contentment and inner peace prevail.

The city was still in the act of awakening when we entered Pathankot; it was then that our driver informed us that he would have to find the agent and pick up our tickets. The exact moment when the cool and laid-back mode of the mountains changed, for we became embroiled in a cloak and dagger mystery affair, and as the driver's stress levels rose, the once clear English-speaker became much harder to understand. Driving frantically up and down the streets and alleyways of the district, stopping folk at street corners, entering shops, jumping out and disappearing down passageways.

And as time moved on towards departure it became clear he was having problems; the driver continued to apologise as he struggled to find the agent. And with empathy rising we told him not to worry, for we would be happy to go back up the big hill, grab another sticky bun, and return to Glenmore.

But so typical of India, and like a flick of the tail of a sacred cow, the scene suddenly changed, the agent materialised waving tickets in hand.

And with the pedal down to the floor we arrived at the

THE DRUID IN THE GREENHOUSE

station just in time to find our names on the carriage sheet, and on boarding and locating our seats, the Pathankot Delhi Express slid away down the side of a bustling platform.

An eight-hour journey to Delhi lay ahead, so once settled it was a case of returning into the laid-back mode of travel, simply observing the passing landscape whilst at times chatting with our fellow passengers.

At station stops along the way, sellers of goods got on and off, a much-appreciated act that helped to shorten the journey.

However, we planned to change at Delhi for another two-and-a-half-hour journey to Agra, and a visit to the Taj Mahal.

On arrival at Delhi station and with a short time to make our connection I had a quick wander around the platform, on passing what appeared to be a second-hand book stand, one little green book caught my attention, it was a sort of 'Hey, I am here waiting for you'. So, without hesitation I had a quick scan of the contents, paid the attendant a few rupees and slipped it into my bag.

Once seated on the train and opening the book, there it was before my eyes, just a few small pages explaining exactually what had happened to me on that fateful day when my head exploded. I had received a massive kundalini awakening, having unknowingly activated the dormant serpent energy that is said to be coiled three and a half times at the base of the spine. The power of nature uniting with that of the universe rose at such a force that it sent me into a state of a spiritual emergency. It was interesting that I discovered this at Diwali, the festival of light, celebrated by the earthly lighting of firecrackers and rockets.

In a time long before Google, gaining knowledge of such things was inaccessible to many, this finding brought about immense relief, a piece in the jigsaw that provided endless scope for further study, and controlled practice. Being someone with a mind to follow the heart and go with the flow of the universe, I understood that the book was there at exactly the right moment when the conscious seeker would arrive.

After a comfortable journey we arrived at Agra station, and being a pair of only a dozen other Westerners we were met by a legion of taxi, rickshaw, and cart driver wallahs. The very ones who appeared willing to enter into civil war to secure our business. Obviously, money was tight and that is a shame, but as you travel throughout India you become exposed to the suffering of all beings, and yet on the turning of a leaf, the hidden flower radiates her beauty.

With that in mind one feels compassion, but as a passing observer in a place where scams abound, there is actually nothing you can do for the masses, yet in a small way, just like here at home, by being conscious you can spot those who remain helpless, where a little assistance may go a long way.

On checking in to our pre-booked hotel at Diwali, the arriving darkness of the day gave rise to a thunderous event, as what seemed like millions of fireworks rising up into the sky, and with increasing explosions reached a crescendo resembling a blitzkrieg. Even whilst sat at the breakfast table next morning the barrage still continued, but the day was intended for sightseeing, and the first call was the Taj Mahal. As we queued and slowly made our way towards the entrance, the excitement generated by the visiting nationals raised the vibration, then on catching a first glimpse we discovered that the Taj was even more magnificent than we could ever have expected. For it stood majestic with a hint of another worldly attitude. Yet it was the embracing feeling of unity with fellow human beings, as we walked together through the peaceful ornamental garden settings, consciously stopping to take in the sight of the feature, the beckoning hand of ivory white marble. For the bulbous central dome of the mausoleum radiates a power and once inside a feeling of joy, simply taking a step back, enthralled at the lattice artwork and an elegance too ornate for me to describe. Like fire merging into air, we absorbed the pleasantness, that radiant joy of the Indian people, who on that special day of their existence came to absorb the power of their cherished national mausoleum of love, a deserving wonder of the world. And after a visit to the Red Fort and a spectacular view of the Taj from the sadly polluted river, we took time out to go shopping, before returning to our hotel. Being located in the Sadar Bazaar area we were only a good walk away from the Zorba the Buddha, an Osho Zoroastrian vegetarian restaurant. I had heard of Osho, but only knew a little of the old Persian religion, in India followers are known as the Parsi, I was aware of the Towers of Silence where the bodies of the dead are left out on the rooftops for disposal by scavenger birds, an ancient practice that I do understand.

It was early evening when we handed in our key at reception, stepped out of the hotel grounds, and headed down to a lane with timber market stalls openly displaying fireworks, and with a wall and narrow pathway it left little room for manoeuvre. After a delicious meal in a laid-back and friendly place, we stepped outside into the darkening evening, joining the hordes of colourfully dressed family members venturing out for an end of day stroll. You could absorb the feel of excitement, humans everywhere, pushing cycles, children at play, young girls and women carrying all manner of wares. But as we ventured into the market stall lane, our minds of peace were changed by the sense of danger, the sight of local men purchasing fireworks for their children, and with plenty in hand enthusiastically bent down and ignited them on the ground directly below the stalls. And as a realm of complete chaos engulfed the lane, we had no other option than to pass through a tunnel of fire safety madness. On reaching our hotel, the high white walls provided some refuge, we watched on as the barrage of ground to air mini missiles were launched into the night sky. After another noisy night in Agra, we travelled to the rail station and boarded a train to the capital city.

Delhi, a seat of grand mastery in the art of scamming, from shoe sprayers to wholesale street actors, silent watchers, and those that approach with helpful guidance, scaremongers and rescuers that lead you to a place of safety, which turns out to be yet another sales trap. But once armed with this knowledge it can be a most experiencing event, a planned walk to a certain place of interest. At first just being aware of the outer watchers, those sets of eyes that observe your every movement, calculating your desire, whilst you continue to play the role of the dumb target. At times it feels that every incoming scam is connected, with game changers and generals pulling at the strings of the unsuspected purse.

Once having skilfully negotiated the scam zone of organised madness and upon nearing the building of your intended visit, the atmosphere changes to one of normality, and for peace of mind's sake you may drop your guard. On arrival a smartly dressed man standing inside the entrance doorway delivers his pleasantries, an in-depth history of the site and the cost of entry. You suddenly feel an inner signal, pick up on a telling glance, maybe a slight mistake of words, and your streetwise awareness rises to the fore once more. Clink, the penny drops, followed by the realisation that he is an end game player, the very one that has had you followed from your hotel, only to be subtly herded like a fellside sheep farmer with his trusted dog.

During your time in India, how you handle this is of great importance. Do you retreat and become timid then submit and open your purse, get angry, scream, shout and front him out, laugh out loud with disrespect, or do you just smile with a level of calmness that informs him politely that you've sussed out his scam, taking your leave with a degree of nobility?

For whilst travelling in India it is cool to remember that with the contact of an eye, one can get anything that you may or may not desire.

A train journey west took us to sample the delights of Jaipur, and after a return bus to New Delhi, two more nights saw our time in India come to an end. The short trip had been successful with numerous experiences like the journey itself, the Diwali evening meal with members of the Tibetan

Government in exile, the Taj Mahal, visiting Mahatma Gandhi's monument and his last place of being, not to mention shaking hands with the Dalai Lama. But the most important one remained the finding of the little book, the one on Kundalini, and the discovery of what had happened to me on that memorable day when the firework exploded inside my head.

On arrival we found the UK under a blanket of deep snow and being scheduled to return to Aberdeen and a chopper flight offshore, it called for a serious change of climate adjustment and mind management.

During this period, I was aware that my spiritual growth had taken on a new meaning, and fortunately the Eastern teachings had provided further knowledge in the workings of mind, karma, and the egoic self.

Throughout the Kundalini experience my desire to seek and gain knowledge had not faltered, signs that the seeds sown in the mud so long ago were now rising stem-like, pushing on up to a greater height where the rays of cascading light shine more brightly. I had gathered information, knowledge of various schools of thought from a host of locations, differing belief systems spanning a time before writing, when oral teachings were the order of the day.

For I had come to love the indigenous systems, those of the Aboriginal folk, the hunter-gatherers and farmers who lived off the land, the ones with their own spirits and systems of integrity. Standing alongside the teachings of Buddha Shakyamuni, Sri Krishna, Jesus of Nazareth, and Gandhi the very ones we would expect to find in the higher realms of the divine beings.

My task was to meld their teachings together as one in a personal system, but to succeed in that goal I would have to remove the inner walls of division, those implanted from birth by the power of male-dominated religions, and that was my quest.

Yet I was not alone, for I remained aware of being guided, and in taking stock, my immediate hurdle was the fact that those major teachings had all come from the East. In contemplation I saw Earth Mother as my British element, although culturally ingrained within me, institutionally she had been transformed into a discredited witch. And with that in mind I turned my attention back to the direction of China and Japan, for both those great nations have ancient spiritual traditions, the Great Way, and it became apparent that the practice of meditation could draw them all together. Being practitioners from the shallow waters of the West, we tend to see martial arts in the main, a physical force, one of self-defence and how quickly a practitioner could dispose of an assailant. And with further development, one advances to weapons, increased numbers of opponents, and with movement of body and sharpness of mind, the breaking of wood, stacks of slates, with the acceptance that occasionally a knuckle or bone may be broken. And it was during this period, that I was keen to further develop my own meditational format, and within that mode of practice I developed a greater feel of flow and movement, a sense of change and shift of energy, being much akin to the elements, and in particular that of air and water.

POLTERGEIST IN THE STAFF HOUSE, AND THE QUEEN'S LODGE

Today Qatar is known as a global gas producer and location of the football world cup, and after discussions with my Scottish-based company, I agreed to accept a position in the then little-known Gulf state.

The new offshore gas field was still in its infancy, and with large numbers of new wells to be drilled and completed, along with the commissioning of offshore platforms and gas transfer facilities the Gulf state provided plenty of international job opportunities. Initially I was rotating from the UK, my work was varied with onshore and offshore operations and it was during that period we moved into a brand-new staff house.

On entry through a high walled garden the building was fine; it had a large lounge with a wide stairway leading up to first-floor bed and bathrooms, and yet it had a strange feel, one that I could not quite put my finger on. I spent the first week in a large rear room with two single beds, but for some reason I could not get a decent night's sleep, and on the nights when another person shared the room, they also experienced the same problem.

During a busy offshore work schedule, I returned back to the staff house and whilst the others were away, I settled into the bedroom at the front of the bad-night-sleep room. After a meal I was shattered and decided on an early night, and as my head touched the pillow I slipped away into unconscious sleep. Sometime later I suddenly became wide awake, which is not uncommon after sessions of working around the clock on a drilling rig. After spending a short time downstairs, I re-entered the bedroom to be taken aback, as three multicoloured transparent tubes of light were visibly moving around in the top corner of the room adjacent to the doorway. They were approximately 10 cm in diameter and up to a metre in length, and they gave off a slight yellow aura, with a hint of sound. Although this vision was a bit startling, I didn't feel threatened by their presence, and being shattered I took the view to just let them get on with it, and I fell back into a deep sleep. Sometime later I was suddenly awakened by the feel of the duvet flying off the bed, and as I clawed my way back into consciousness my first thoughts were that someone had just played a prank on me. But on opening my eyes I saw that the entire room was now full of the transparent coloured tubes, they were moving in motion as though alive, and on seeing my duvet laid on the floor midway to the doorway I rose to go and retrieve it. On standing and taking the first step I suddenly felt a strong blow to the centre of my back, it was very much like a punch; I instinctively spun around and reacted with a loud *Kiai* as I delivered a controlled punch and kick routine down the unseen line of the hit, upon delivery all the coloured tubes instantly disappeared, and on retrieving my quilt got back into bed, and the room became still once more.

This was not the first time I had taken such action with unfriendly spirit forces, and I knew from experience that they do not respond well to a single-pointed controlled responsive action from a physical being. On another occasion whilst stopping the night in a first-floor room of an old English inn, I encountered a bedroom experience of some similarity. In fact, in those places spirit forces of a various nature are not at all uncommon. But be aware as a more powerful force may stand its ground, and you may well require a different response to bring about its removal. 'It's horses for courses,' whispered the long-deceased stable boy.

But today I still know little of the coloured tubes, with poltergeist being a collective description. On the morning after the flying duvet incident, I received a call to head back offshore, so I booked myself out for an evening departure on a rig support vessel. I enjoyed the experience of being allowed to sit alone outside at the back of the boat, and with the warmth of the breeze I felt grateful for having the opportunity to take in the moment. And as the curtain of the darkness came down to the sea, I sat and contemplated the previous night's events. On arrival at the rig, I discussed my duvet experience with a couple of the lads who shared the staff house, they were due to fly back to the beach that afternoon. As expected, they were amazed by the story, but as usual in cases like this, they remained sceptical, but they did agree that something was not right in that area of the new building.

A few days later when the lads returned to the rig, one appeared to be in a state of shock. He revealed that he had been exposed to a similar experience inside the same bedroom. That he had suddenly awakened when his duvet cover was pulled off the bed And like most people, he quickly scarpered straight out of the bedroom, so at least he never received a blow, and that can only be a good thing. After the offshore work was completed and upon landing back onshore, I returned to the staff house to collect my belongings, then took a flight home. I never had the chance to stay over in that house again, and a short time later our company gave up the lease, so whoever took over residency of the property, my thoughts go out to you.

The situation changed once again when I took up a family position in Qatar. Living in Doha within an expat community can be rewarding, with most people willing to assist one another in a manner of decades past. But it was the communal suffering that I found most fascinating when the news broke that Diana, Princess of Wales, and her partner Dodi Fayed, a film producer and son of Egyptian billionaire Mohamed Al Fayed, had both died in a car crash in Paris. But it was not just the British and Arab communities who felt the loss, for that morning I received numerous calls and the wrapping of arms from people of all nations who were genuinely affected. And as lines of people gathered at the British embassy to sign their names in the book of condolence, the energy created was there to be felt.

It was interesting to observe how that sudden death had instantaneously created such an atmosphere, one of coming together as one people of one nation, called planet Earth. Sadly, it was only to last for a couple of days, before the energy changed, and the lines of division appeared in the sand once more.

Apart from responding to worldly events, living in the Gulf provided business and leisure opportunities, and after a short evening flight to Cairo, we cleared arrivals and took a cab to the Windsor Hotel. On arrival we discovered a place with atmosphere, a quirky one-time British Officers' Club that still radiated a colonial feel. And being tucked away in a tight street of cafés with outside tables and shisha pipe service, it proved a good choice for a four-night stay.

After breakfast we set off to visit the museum of antiquity and whilst slowly wandering the halls we gazed with amazement at the sheer scale of the collection. Artefacts of all shapes and sizes that appeared to have just been dropped on the floor awaiting future siting, and being a day with few people about, it provided a window for a period of contemplation beside the royal mummies. After a couple more days visiting the pyramids, the outdoor markets and the old city mosque, spiritual batteries were well and truly recharged.

Armed with new literature of learning and inspired to delve deeper into Isis, the goddess of love, healing, magic, and the moon, we took the return flight back to Doha. Whilst living in Doha I aggravated a long-time groin injury, one that had first occurred when miskicking a tennis ball in the old school yard.

And along with a martial art mindset of working through injuries, and with the ongoing practice of attempting to achieve the full lotus position, I had not done myself any favours. But help was around the corner when I was introduced to a Chinese doctor, who having exposed me to acupuncture and further healing methods, stated that unfortunately the actions of my past had caught up with me. The extent of my injury meant that my days of sitting in the lotus position were for now somewhat restricted. Apart from his shared knowledge on healing, and conduit energy throughout the body, it was his teachings of the soft style tai chi that left me inspired.

During our stay in Doha my daughter worked as a cabin crew member for Qatar Airways, a position that allowed the family to purchase cheap flight tickets, and with Nepal just over five hours flight away, it provided an opportunity that could not be missed. It was late November when we entered the airport's departure lounge for a night-time flight to Kathmandu, and on entry we were pleasantly surprised to find the place full of hikers who had arrived off a connecting flight from Heathrow. After a delay in departing and a sleepy night flight with the first rays of the sun penetrating the darkness, the aircraft banked over as it made its way cautiously around the hillside of the Kathmandu Valley. A closeness that provided a view and a feeling that you could almost say 'Namaste' to the awakening people in the houses below. Due to work commitments, we only had a short visit, so with a mind to make the most of what was on offer, we hurriedly left departures and made our way to the Thamel district, an area of the city that caters mostly for

THE DRUID IN THE GREENHOUSE

the Western visitor, and it did not take long to find a suitable place to stay, a hotel run by a friendly Tibetan family. It was during the first day of wandering the tightly packed smoky and vibrant streets, that on the turning of a corner I walked straight into my past, a shock to the system. For right there, hanging on a wall before me, were the faces of the ones who used to visit my Lancashire bedroom some 40 years previous. And on recovering from the initial shock, investigations revealed they were Dharmapala masks, those of powerful deities, bearing wrathful expressions, the ones worn by the tribal shaman in ritual during the practices of healing, for exorcisms and other purposes. And the question now was, how and why had they come to visit me on numerous occasions? And if I was to ask a local man of knowledge, he may have informed me that, in a past life, I too would have worn the mask. And on reflection, I was happy with that.

During our visit we met up with a couple of friends from the UK who were trekking in the area, and after a few days visiting local sites like the Great Stupa at Boudhanath, and the Monkey Temple with its splendid views, three of us arranged with a local driver to take us on a day out. Our chosen destination was a couple of hours drive away, and on arrival found it to be located in a wooded hillside setting where monkeys roamed in abundance.

Vajrayogini Temple, a Tibetan Buddhist Tantric deity whom at the time I studied and worked with, and on arrival, it had a feeling that we were expected. The Nepalese are the loveliest of people that you could ever wish to meet, but for me, within their culture lies a practice of wrongdoing, and that is the sacrificing of live animals, and I wish and pray that they would stop, Namaste. On arrival back in Qatar, the topographical features and cultural differences between them and Nepal are a paradigm shift that at times can prove difficult to adjust, but what goes on within is the true yardstick. As a seeker of knowledge, the discovery of the Dharmapala masks had been one of significance, for that shamanic connection had provided me with an avenue for greater research; and along with the visit to the Vajrayogini Temple proved it was a living place, and not just something practised from a book. As the universe revealed its secrets the years of dedication to practise within a mishmash of belief systems continued to slip into place.

After months of being spiritual awakened by the early morning calls to prayer from the local muezzin, we arrived at Sri Lanka's international airport.

And due to recent incidents involving the ongoing troubles between the government and the Tamil Tigers, the place was in a bit of a lockdown mode.

After some time spent clearing arrivals, we managed to jump onto a southbound bus for a journey down to the west coast resort of Hikkaduwa. We found a nice room inside a walled garden that backed onto the sea, a lovely spot that I fear may well have been destroyed in the Boxing Day 2004 tsunami. After a few days of chilling in the local beach cafés, wandering around the old Portuguese and since fortified Dutch fort at Galle, the time came to move on.

After an early breakfast we travelled north to visit the preserved ruins at the ancient sites in the Anuradhapura district, the northern region was still a Tamil Tiger war zone, but with a wave of our passports and a friendly smile, the checkpoint soldiers raised the barriers and allowed us to pass through.

It was late morning when we arrived at a Lakeside Lodge.

Upon enquiring about vacancies, the manager nervously informed us that he only had one room left, and as we were British, we may like the room that our Queen and Prince Philip once stayed in during their 1954 royal visit to the then named Ceylon. It was then that I noticed a strange reaction from a member of staff, he was given a key and instructions to show me the room.

On following him down a corridor of bedrooms we came to a lobby with a separate door. On entry it was quite a large room, containing two single four-poster beds draped with mosquito nets, the rear had a lounge seating area and a set of patio doors. Upon opening it led to a landing stage with private boat access to the large lake, one that provided water-level views across to the distant wooded shoreline. The walls of the room housed a number of framed old black and white photos of the Queen and Prince Philip, taken during their stay at the purpose-built lodge. The collection included pics of their time spent out on the lake, and along with the original furniture of that period it seemed a fine place to spend a few days. Having informed the senior member of staff that we would take the room for three nights, he seemed surprised, and repeated that since our queen

THE DRUID IN THE GREENHOUSE

had stayed there, it should be OK for us.

Obviously, something was not right, but with a lack of further options, we checked in with positive minds. Once unpacked we decided to go out for a walk down the road to a place that we observed had a cycle for hire sign. The area had a canal/river system with numerous paths and with ancient sites all within cycling distance, it seemed a promising idea.

After a 15-minute walk we came to a farm-like set-up, and apart from bike rentals it had a café with an outside seating area. Having viewed the menu and placed our order, we settled in for a relaxing lunch.

But the atmosphere of peace suddenly changed, when a friendly cockerel came over to say hello; instantly a mature man came running out of the building shouting and screaming and with a kick, sent the poor bird sprawling into the adjoining table and chairs. Without hesitation I instinctively jumped up and confronted the man who turned out to be the owner; my actions had caught him by surprise and he nervously stated that he was angry the bird had come over to annoy his paying guests. After explaining that we had no problem with the cockerel and with some further discussion on cruelty, cause and effect, the situation calmed. The owner returned with a luncheon of delights, and in conversation he asked where we were staying. When I informed him, we were staying in the lodge, he responded by asking if we were staying in the in the Queen's Room, on confirmation, he appeared startled, and even though I pushed him he ignored my request to explain.

Over lunch we discussed how bizarre and mixed-up things

had actually become when two Westerners were less afraid of spirit forces than the locals, who then ended up explaining the effect of wrong actions to the people of a Buddhist /Hindu society. But on analysing I realised that being a Western seeker of spiritual knowledge in a land where it is taught from birth, I had actually misjudged how strong the effects of the civil war conflict must have had on their daily lives. Also, something was obviously wrong with our room; the locals all appeared too scared to explain. Did it have anything to do with the queen who had stayed there five decades ago, or had something else happened there since, had acts of horror and death occurred inside the room? Having rode back to the lodge we settled in for a mid-afternoon siesta. The room felt a bit odd, but nothing like the cold, dark and scary environment that appeared to be on the midnight menu. We spent the rest of the afternoon cycling along the waterside lanes, a chilled mode, taking in the delights of the flora and fauna, which included huge water monitors, a place where locals asked if we were Dutch.

We returned to the lodge for evening dinner and after sampling the delights of a vegetarian meal, we returned to the room. Darkness was rapidly descending as we spent the final minutes of light stood out on the landing stage absorbing the moment. The feel of the lake setting, the breeze on our faces, those smells, and the sounds of splashing out on the vast water, the repeated call of communication between roost-seeking birds, as darting bats took their places in the beckoning night sky. Returning inside we lit some incense and settled down to chill in the once regal setting. However, it was only a matter of minutes before swirling shapes of light appeared around the entrance door wall area, whilst at the opposite end they came into view at the patio doors. We motioned to each other as the room began to fill with shapes of light that moved towards and all around us, and as time went on some of the shapes turned figure-like and continued to move around the room in a manner likened to the images we later saw inside Hogwarts' dining room. Although it was a full-on visual display neither of us felt scared, and at times were amazed by their size and movement as the evolving figure shapes danced and became one with the drifting smoke of incense. I was half expecting a scary finale but that never came, and to the best of my knowledge the show went on for most of the night, but once day light returned the room became the norm once more.

At the breakfast table next morning, the manager with lurking staff members within earshot, asked us if we managed to get a good night's sleep. On saying we did, and on making a reference to the ghostly figures, he went into a bit of a panic mode, and whilst scurrying away repeated that it was good to have people from the queen's homeland staying in the room. The following day was spent visiting the ancient sites whilst the events of the second night were similar to the first, and by the third night the visions increased to a crescendo. The entire room became full of the ghostly shapes, homing in through the mosquito nets with increased force, before swerving away or sliding around our faces. In fact, in the end, it became a bit boring, or maybe they were building up for a fourth night extravaganza, on that we will never know. At checkout the next day, one of the staff nervously informed me that previous guests had ran out during the first night, and that no one would ever stay in that room, admitting they were all amazed that we had lasted three nights. Having left the area to visit the Sigiriya rock fortress and the amazing Dambulla cave temple, we spent the last few days of the trip staying in a lovely bungalow overlooking the sacred lake at Kandy.

But unfortunately, the monsoon had arrived a good month early; we spent our last car journey heading down the road in a torrential downpour. In fact, it was so bad that to our left trees and sections of the mountainside could be seen sliding down towards us, and down to our right a swollen river with flowing cars rushed on by. Our driver excitedly pointed and laughed as we pushed on down the mountain road to arrive safely in the city of Colombo.

BAREFOOTING ON THE SANDS OF NEW BEGINNINGS

It was the third day of the new millennium, and with an ardent desire for a period of freedom, we obtained two flight tickets, and with little planning, embarked on a journey to the southern Indian state of Kerala.

Our intention was to find a place to rent for a couple of months or so, visit the Western Ghats, then cross over to the east and follow the coastline up to Kolkata, before heading north to the tea plantations, and the Himalayan state of Sikkim.

Similar to Sri Lanka, Kerala's economy relies on the exportation of labour to the Arabian Gulf states. But unlike our experience, theirs can be somewhat cruel, for on arrival at Thiruvananthapuram Airport, young mothers having signed up to work for months or even years can be seen wailing and shedding tears as they drudgingly shuffle their way to the departure lounge. Others can be seen with faces tight against tear-stained windows, as older relatives on the opposite side hug their children, and as the curtain came down on the final act of eternal love, we humbly passed by. Being a witness to this emotional exchange of near helplessness can be quite disturbing, and to the eye of a Western mind a stark reminder to the rawness of suffering that these people are raised to endure. Struck by silence, and on the turning of a card, we made our way to the arrival's hall, and out into the midday sun.

After a few days relaxing in a small rice field chalet, we embarked on a mission to find a place to rent, and after a couple of days searching, found a suitable property, agreed on a price, and moved into a two bedroomed bungalow.

A lovely, detached whitewashed building with terracotta roof tiles, hidden below the coconut trees with an outside staircase providing access to a flat-roofed area, and with a raised seated veranda that overlooked the beautiful flora of the white-walled garden, we settled in nicely, thank you. Our new home was in a valley and being only a twenty-minute walk down to the beachside amenities, it provided the best of both worlds.

The immediate neighbours kept chickens and allowed us to purchase up to two newly laid eggs every other day, a hut stall at the top road sold milk, yogurt, bread, and local vegetables, and with a bus stop across the road it provided the means for a weekly shopping trip into the city of Thiruvananthapuram.

A Christian church occupied the plot at the rear of the walled garden, and on occasions whilst sat sampling the stunning evening setting, the enthusiastic congregation delivered a rousing session of music and song. One of the main attractions for Westerners was the Ayurvedic treatment centres, where groups of mainly ladies would arrive to learn about its concepts and healing practices, and on gaining knowledge and skills returned home to offer their treatments to those in need. It was the beginning of January and in southern India the afternoons are hot, and after the initial holiday mode had started to wane, the slowing-down process began. Longer siestas became the norm, providing a window to spend a few hours each day reading, meditating, and in contemplation, it started to have an effect. For that oscillating state of toing and froing had ceased, and I became aware of distinct images of people from my past experiences. In fact, a complex mode of memory that brought back situations where I had been harmful and unkind, an emotional process that gave rise to feelings of guilt, shame, and embarrassment, and also from the other way, where persons had been unkind to me. Although alarmingly exposed to the realities of my past actions, I was aware that by allowing a deeper connection to manifest, it would enhance my spiritual awakening. And with plenty of time on my side I decided to go with a project, and with a little bit of mind management and with the aid of mediation techniques, I began to analyse the whole of my life so far. Having first stated my intentions, it took over, for I was shown images, one's going right back to the cradle of this lifetime, incidents, recollections, things said or done that had caused harm to others. Sitting down and watching a video of your own life can be alarming, for being exposed to the clarification of my behaviour, a re-run of the early crafting's of manipulation against my own parents, my friends and others, and the acceptance that those actions still had an effect on me and others to this day. But the process was not just about people I had known or met, it went much deeper, with faces and places of brief encounters: the man I was rude to in a bank doorway entrance, the conflict with the conductress when I jumped on her moving bus, forcefully pushing the cat off my seat. And as the days and weeks went by, I slowly sifted through the growing pile of re-encountered events. In fact, more or less every person I had ever met or made contact.

After the sessions I took time to work through the experiences, keeping records, analysing, reliving those happenings, and although I saw the wrongs of others, it was my wrongdoings that I felt compelled to concentrate on. And on completion apologising to all those I had harmed or disrespected, and yet it never felt right to ask for forgiveness. It became a realisation that everything thing we do, every action we make, including our thoughts will have an effect, and I went into a period of self-healing, and I came out of this chapter of life feeling very humble.

It was around a decade or so later that my path of the seeker took me to the place of the lightworker, where I was informed that the process, I went through in Kerala takes place after death. For after leaving the physical body and the elements behind, with a change of vibrational energy, the soul is required to go through a process of healing. One that includes exposure to a re-run of its past life experiences. In summary the time spent reliving my present life was a significant event, one that left me consciously aware of my future actions, including those of my rising thoughts, thus leaving me with the task of having a greater respect for every living thing, all forms of existence.

But life was kind, and some evenings, we would wander

along the paths of the coconut forest and down to the beach huts for evening dinner. On rare occasions my daughter and her cabin crew mates would meet up and gather around large tables, and as the curtain of darkness fell small crabs would crawl out from the sand beneath our feet, raising reactions from the unsuspecting crew members.

Being nestled nicely by the side of the fruitful Arabian Sea provides a constant stream of seafood that arrived daily in the form of fresh shellfish, swordfish, redfish and tuna, the ones the beach hut chefs turn into interesting delicacies. However, the catch of the day was not always a constant, as it relied upon the skills and good fortunes of the local fishermen. Some mornings I would rise early and go for a walk along the seashore, for me the period just after sunrise remains the best time of day. A group of four or five fishermen were usually active, and I sometimes stayed around long enough to watch them cast their exceptionally large nets. It was a process achieved by leaving one section of the roped net on the steepish sandy beach, as men in a plank-built boat and a dugout canoe began paying out the net, as they rowed out to sea. And I can confirm they went out an exceptionally long way, for with eyes pinched you could just about make them out, as they bobbed up and down on the swell of the ocean.

It was mid-morning, the sky was clear, a soft warm breeze stroked the senses, and in the setting of a tune from The Art of Noise, without a care I strolled along the shoreline barefooted. And as the pull of the ebbing tide gently rolled and fell away, it captured the felt rhythm of the sound of the moment.

But the day was suddenly brought into play, for like a cleaning cloth rubbed over smeared spectacles, the peace of the occasion was wiped away.

Far along the beach to the north, I observed an unusual commotion, and I took the decision to take a closer look. After a good walk I arrived and entered a scene of the like I had not previously witnessed, for before me stood a line of local men agonisingly pulling on the end of the rope, whilst the two men about 200 metres out in the boats were shouting and signalling with hand movements. At this point, a group of around a dozen Western tourists had gathered to watch the proceedings, and as the noise levels increased more local men arrived to offer support to the struggling rope pullers. I had previously observed the fishermen haul in their nets, but this time it was different, and I only realised the scale of the difference when two men ran past me, plunged into the water, and began to swim out towards the boats. And as the two sets of men on the steep sandy beach continued to pull, the buoys on the gathering net came into view. There was a lot of high-pitched excited Malayalam exchanged between the boatmen and those in the water. One of the swimmers turned around and headed back to the beach; he rose from the water shouting in English: 'Big fish, many big fish.' At this point more local men arrived to assist, the atmosphere became very intense, and as the two boats neared the shoreline the loop in the large net began to close, large, trapped tuna started to leap up into the air, with one managing to escape over the side net. Amazingly in order to confuse the fish three men ran into the netted area started to splash around, and as the men on the beach pulled on the ropes in unison, the loop tightened. Apart from everything else I became concerned for the welfare of the men in the water, for they were not only putting themselves at risk of being harmed by the power of a fish, but they could get caught up inside the net and drown. And as the pullers gradually heaved the net up onto the steep sandy beach, the water came alive, boiling with frantic attempts to escape. And with a final pull, the end of the net appeared to reveal a pod, a family of tuna, and as the larger males and females began leaping high in the air, they came crashing down on the hard sand, as their babies flapped on.

Dark blood poured out onto the once golden sand, the gasps and screams of horror from the Western tourists filled the once peaceful setting, and even the local men who had simply come to assist were in shock as the fisherman frantically attempted to cudgel the struggling huge fish to death.

As I watched on consciously praying for them to die quickly, it continued for far too long before the last of the flapping ceased. And as the final moment arrived, every one of us, including the fishermen stood together in silence, and with heads down and eyes fixed, in unity we became immersed in a deep sense of guilt. Genocide came to mind, we had just witnessed the slaughter of a pod of 20 animals, ranging in sizes from 5 feet adults down to 1.5 feet of the young.

Although obviously delighted by the size of the catch the fishermen still showed remorse and were genuinely aware of the discomfort that their actions had had on the tourists. For it opened the door to death itself, the bodies lying there on the beach could well have been human, for the sight of beings suffering at the end of life brings no distinctions. With respect the group of tourists turned and slowly walked away in a manner reserved for a funeral, and as I gazed into the eyes of the two nearest fishermen, they showed deep remorse, somewhat ashamed, but they too have to survive, to live, to feed and support their own families. And as I turned to walk the mile back down the isolated seashore, it felt like the world itself had changed, a crack in humanity, nothing will ever be the same again; my thoughts were of forgiveness to a greater power, as 'Anthem' by Leonard Cohen supported the turntable of contemplation.

Living in a land below the coconut palms, where every part of the bountiful tree is used to sustain human life, whether a floor covering, body and hair oil or simply an alcoholic toddy, can at times be dangerous. For as the nuts mature, they became heavy, and during our stay we were awakened to the sound of nut-laden branches crashing down upon the building's flat roof, not to mention the visiting large spiders, an appearance that did not go down too well when our daughter arrived to find a furry friend had taken up residence in her shower. Her arrival spurred us on to book seats on a day's bus excursion into Tamil Nadu and down to the holy town of Kanyakumari/Cape Comorin located at the southern tip of India. Recognised as a place of spiritual importance where Gandhi's ashes were immersed in the sea, when on a particular day you can experience the sun setting and the moon rising simultaneously over the ocean. During a full moon in spring, the Chitra Pournami, an auspicious day

THE DRUID IN THE GREENHOUSE

for erasing old karma, for when the sun is exalted in Aries with the moon in Libra, devotees gather to invoke Chitragupta, the bookkeeper of karmic records.

Unfortunately, we were a few months short, but still found the place buzzing with excited families as they rushed to bathe within the ebb and flow of the crashing waves. After a long day sightseeing, we returned to the bus stand and on arrival back in Thiruvananthapuram we found a large political rally underway with thousands of brightly dressed individuals swelling the streets, and after a run and a jump onto a departing bus, we arrived back home.

A few hours later the cockerels of the neighbourhood informed us that another sunny day lay ahead, and the first stroll out revealed new colourful advertisements placed on walls and posts. Upon further scrutiny they pronounced a date when the local community were holding a festival event where martial arts and traditional costumed dancers would perform.

With tickets purchased in advance, the day of the event came around, and as we made our way downhill the route was highlighted with numerous colourful sheets secured to trees by long ropes, elemental characters emerged as they moved and fluttered in motion with the warm sea breeze.

On presenting our tickets we were channelled down a sandy entrance pathway where friendly ushers directed us towards part sand buried seats, and on passing the stage I was taken back, in fact, slightly shocked. For their standing before me were a group of figures wearing head masks that bore a resemblance to those worn by my bedroom visitors all those years ago.

As the performances commenced, I was particularly interested in the southern Indian martial art of Kalaripayattu, which like those of the Chinese styles came into prominence through observing the fighting techniques of wild animals, in this case that of the crocodile, which to my observation would come into its own, once one had been grounded.

Our time in Kerala concluded when we obtained train tickets for an evening departure to Tamil Nadu, and the holy pilgrim city of Madurai.

After ten weeks of being at one with land, sea, and sky, with a touch of sadness, we said goodbye to the neighbours, threw on our rucksacks, nodded to the gathering hens, crossed the road, and embarked on our final bus journey.

'Walkin' My Cat Named Dog', a quirky folky early R&B number by Norma Tenega, came to mind.

On arrival at the rail station, we settled down on a welcoming bench, with daylight receding the platform lights provided a comforting feel, and with time to spare we reflected on the experience so far, the present situation, and what lay ahead. For me there is no greater feeling of aliveness, than pulling on a rucksack, tightening the money belt, and with passport and a ticket set off on an adventure to an unknown place.

Being the first of many planned sleeper train journeys, we knew little of the procedures or what to expect, and the first thing we learnt was that notices bearing your names and seat numbers are posted on the outside of each carriage. And with each long seat becoming a bunk, an enthusiastic young man made his way down the carriage handing out packs of clean

THE DRUID IN THE GREENHOUSE

bedding. The train journeys are a miniature version of Indian life, and in order to handle and enjoy, just consciously slip into a chill mode, and with a sense of just being happy to be alive, simply go with the flow. Being an avid lifelong train-traveller and a person that has developed a view that we are simply here to experience, it is how we handle it that affects what comes next. For I do appreciate that sleeper trains across India, especially those journeys of over 30 hours in length, where you may go to bed twice, eat numerous meals, along with the need to visit the toilets, are not in keeping with the views of most Western folk. The saying 'Each to their Own' may suffice. After an interesting night of rocking, sleeping, and awakening to the strange sounds from within and without, the carriage suddenly became alive when a man with meaningfulness came through the carriage shouting chai and vegetable cutlets. As another collected our spent bed rolls, it signalled the start of a new day of delightful, organised chaos. With fellow passengers arising from slumber, it resembled a scene from music festivals past, and after a quick visit to the loo with toothbrush in hand, a splash of cold water and a flick from a cleansing wipe, we sat back to enjoy our food and drink.

After a period of jolts, stops, and starts, daylight arrived and through the barred windows came the sights of an awakening India. And with the first gaze of the day, out in the fields folk were taking their morning ablutions, buffalo wandered as egrets fished, when a man came down the carriage to inform us that we were nearing our destination, and within the time it took to burn an incense stick, the train slowly came to a halt at Madurai junction. We had plans for a three-night stay and having pre-booked a hotel by telephone, we trundled away in a rickshaw, and in no time at all checked into our clean, but sparse room.

Madurai is a pilgrim city, and the hotel played its part when the highlight of the day arrived with the ringing of a loud bell, a sound that alerted the guests that the adjacent temple's painted elephant had arrived with its eager mahout.

On leaning over the first-floor balcony wall with a rupee note in hand, a searching trunk quickly whisked it away and into the clutches of the smiling collector, something different when likened to a *Big Issue* street vendor with trusted dog. Madurai is one of southern India's oldest cities, with its main attraction being the enormous Sri Meenakshi Temple, a breathtaking example of Dravidian architecture with its towering multicoloured images of gods and goddesses, with mythical creatures bearing down from all directions. After removing our shoes, we made our way inside a place that resembled a huge cavern, and with its sanctuaries and many shrines attracts hordes of pilgrims and visitors from a far. For me it was a place that heightened the senses, sights of mystical colourful shapes, as people in all manner of costumes passed us by, but it was not just the sights, but the smells of elephant, incense, and the fragrance of marigolds. Deities, the sound of mantras chanted, prayers of devotion uttered and spoken, drifting smoke, splashes of water and the tinkling of bells. And for hours, with every step of bare foot laid on stone, we wandered unnoticed.

After a few days of intensive happenings, it was time to seek peace and solitude, and after an early rise we boarded a bus for the three-and-a-half-hour journey up to the Western Ghats, and the hill station of Kodaikanal.

Kodai is a place of outstanding beauty and at an altitude of 2,100 metres it can rain a lot. In fact, on checking into a room in a Yorkshire style cottage, the mist was so thick you could hardly see, and so it remained for three days.

On the fourth we rose to find that the rain had ceased, the mist had cleared, and with a bright sun shining; it came as a shock to find the view from our window offered the essence of a sublime vista. Apart from a respite from the heat of the plains the small town had plenty to offer, with a good choice of eateries, like the popular Tibetan Brothers, and after a good walk a delicious evening meal at the Manna bakery. The town had lakesides to wander, and as honeymoon couples took to boating, the walks in the nearby hills paid homage to the mother of sheer beauty, for the sights and smells of fruit trees, an abundance of flowers in springtime bloom, energised the souls of our being.

After a few more days of wandering, getting into discussions with local philosophers, just simply absorbing the energy of place, the time to move on sadly came around. Having visited a local agency, we managed to purchase two sleeper tickets on a 1am train to Chennai, and with the nearest station Kodai Road a 50-mile bus ride away, it provided ample time for thought. For it is at times like this when you may realise just how vulnerable you actually are. For on alighting the bus at the rail station, appearing to be in the middle of nowhere, shrouded in darkness, with a three hour wait, we sat alone at the end of a long platform. And with the inviting sounds of Indian pop music drifting across from a neighbouring village coming to an end, most of the lights went out.

Sitting all alone in a strange land, the sight of small groups of men with an occasional pair crossing the rails, walking the platform to check us out, kept us alert. For one has to send out the right vibrations, an aura of protection, and at such times it is also good to remember that they don't know who you are, and that remains your advantage. Our destination, the east coastal town of Mahabalipuram, and with its famous shore temple, a place where Western travellers choose to gather. In fact, we had pre-arranged to meet up with two friends from the UK who were making their way over from Sri Lanka. Apart from the chillout zone of the town, two neighbouring places of interest were the French-influenced town of Pondicherry and Kanchipuram, one of the seven holy cities of India. And after a week of wandering around and sampling the local delicacies, a bus trip to Kanchipuram made its way to the top of list. After an early start and on acquiring two seats on a local bus the huge gopurams of the 125 remaining temples came into view. And on climbing down from the rickety vehicle the place was alive with masses of pilgrims; many were gathering at the gates of the main Sri Ekambaranathar Temple. A place of Shiva the destroyer, worshipped as a lingam, one who some Western travellers view as a Bob Marley-type figure, who along with Brahma and Vishnu form the Hindu trinity. And on realising that we were the only Western folk in sight that day, experience had taught us that when the usual demands from an assortment of men came our way, we would have to remain direct in our actions.

Most temples in India allow non-Hindus access, you may have to pay a few rupees to enter, a camera fee, cover your bare legs and remove your flip-flops and sandals. But we crossed words with a temple Brahmin when we did not take up his request to pay an extra fee to have our more expensive footwear looked after, instead much preferring to place them inside our daily use backpacks. He then informed me I could not enter because I was wearing a top, and when I pointed out that most other men were wearing shirts, I realised that a payment to look after our invisible shoes was the only way to gain entry. Flagging after a full morning of walking the site, the idea of a drink and lunch brought much interest. Having rested in the shade, we set off on a cool rickshaw ride to the gates of the Devarajaswami, the Temple of Vishnu, a deity known as the preserver and protector of the universe in Hindu tradition.

The holy Temple of Vishnu is a huge high-walled site, with towering gopurams and elaborate stone carvings that become enhanced by the pouring of light rays from the afternoon sun. And like all visits to temple towns and cities, you come to a point when you just cannot absorb anymore, and with that realisation we climbed into a rickshaw and headed back to the bus station. After a hot and sticky return journey to Mahabalipuram, we arrived back in our cool room, and after the taking of showers, followed by an evening meal, brought a close to an interesting day.

After a couple more days spent relaxing and just wandering around town without purpose, the way pointed to Pondicherry, a former French colony that was only a good bus ride away. This time three of us took to the road, and as the journey headed south past sweeping sands where hardly anyone seemed to venture, that feel of something new filtered through. On arrival we discovered a city of two halves, a place where the India of today embraces the old French colonial past, and with a quarter displaying whitewashed architecture and a cuisine to match, it brought a pleasant change. One of the remarkable things that came out of the visit was the feeling of the freshness of the promenade, with its stalls and cafés, and a Victorian-like pier where the coolness of the ocean swept in with an aura of regal dignity. On personal reflection this period in India was having an effect, for when moving around the country I had noticed that the local dogs were taking an interest in me.

It had started back in Kerala when they appeared at my side in ones and twos, and again in Kodaikanal where the small group of street dogs would observe, rise, and cross the road to walk behind me, it was all so light-hearted that we even gave some names. But on arrival at more populated places, they came up and stared, before following. But of course, in India nothing goes unnoticed by the eye of the watcher, Pondicherry was no different, maybe even a highlight, for once the tide had receded, we went for a stroll on the sandy beach. During our slow return from the low-water mark a large pack of dogs who had been asleep by the pier glanced over, and as the big bruiser of many fights rose up and walked towards us the rest did follow. For me this gave rise to a tinge of embarrassment, for I had only recently noticed that the street bulls and cows were starting to act in the similar manner. But I was taken aback, when the pack of about 15 dogs tucked in behind their leader and proceeded to follow me up the beach. Feeling a bit edgy I stopped and turned to witness a sea of furry faces. I would have loved to have produced food and fresh water, all laid out and presented in individual bowls, alas, just like the other half lives. But on turning and striding I became conscious of the big leader closing the gap between us, and in doing so he licked my hand. Strangely I took his action as a bit of an honour, although the threat of the spread of disease immediately came to mind. I said hello and smiled back with some appreciation. They continued to follow us off the beach when a local man approached and standing before me stated that he had been watching the behaviour of the dogs, and on offering his hand to mine, looked into my eyes, and said, 'Sir, you have a true gift,' and on holding my hand bowed his head in reverence. An act of pure India that I truly love. And yes, I was embarrassed by his claim, but I was aware that I was giving off a level of vibration that the animals adhered to, and he wasn't the last man in India to approach me. Being in a place where anything is possible, I had no idea where this could be taking me, and as a visitor with no one to turn to for guidance, I took to playing it down. About the same time, I became aware of a place not so far away, where one could go to have not just your charts read, but they would actually inform you of the exact date and how your death would occur. Although it may sound a bit scary, it still had a power of fascination, and with a little investigation I discovered it wasn't somewhere you could just turn up and pay a fee, but quite the opposite. Although at the time I didn't follow it up, on returning to the UK, I did gain further knowledge of the subject.

But for the Westerner, the main attraction and reason for visiting Pondicherry is the place of 'The Mother' named Auroville, a spiritual village where international men and woman can come together to live in peace and harmony. We found the village in a lovely setting near to the sea, and after a pleasant walk from the bus stand entered the main reception, and on checking out what was on offer, we decided to book in for the day. And in doing we were committed to a change of clothing, although similar, a different colour to those worn by longer-term residents. After wandering around the lovely gardens, we entered the community shop, a place that sold scarfs, bags, books, and quality incense that nowadays are available for purchase in a range of UK outlets. On leaving the shop we were informed of an early evening meditation session being held in the inner chamber of the nearly built Matrimandir.

At the time of construction, the building resembled a sort of spacecraft-cum-giant-golf-ball structure, and when the call came to make our way, other groups of people began to make an appearance. Upon walking along a peaceful pathway, we fell into an orderly line, and within the motion of movement towards the sphere, from my right came the pull of an ancient power, a pulsating energy, a call from a large banyan tree.

As we moved onwards, I did feel a little uncomfortable yet remained intrigued, but as the object of the exercise was one of meditation, I would have preferred to nestle beside the inviting tree. But we are here on planet Earth to experience, and on arrival at the entrance to the Matrimandir were greeted by officials, who after a few words, slipped passes over our heads and pointed the way to a spiralling staircase. As we climbed it brought back a memory of queuing to enter the top section of the Statue of Liberty, so many moons before. On arrival at the top of the dome, guides were on hand to show us the way. Following others who had been there before, we moved slowly around the large room in a 'clockwise' direction before taking our places on mats laid out upon the floor. It was all very futuristic, and as waves of ear-calming music filled the air, I sat and observed the chambers central main feature, that of a large crystal globe. After everyone had settled, a man came to the fore; he informed us of the purpose of place before directing us into a 15-minute meditation session. Although a box-ticking experience, on rising and descending the metal stairway, it was the stepping out into the lovely earthly setting that left me with a feeling of arriving by craft from elsewhere. On returning down the pathway the old banyan tree waved, so I took the opportunity to go over and pay my respects, for if a living tree was good enough for Buddha Shakyamuni, then it certainly was for me.

Trees, the standing people, it is an interesting thought that like humans, a tree naturally starts life as a seed and over time grows up to become a magnificent form of being, and much like us is subjected to the power of the elements and adapts its life accordingly. Some trees may be fortunate to live out their lives in a lovely setting, maybe an old churchyard or the side of a delightful valley, and with ample water and sunlight providing a home for numerous other creatures. And like many of us, other trees are far less fortunate, starting their lives growing up in a tight and compact community, vying for space on a dense woodland floor, stunted, deformed, and twisted as they seek out the light. It may well be the wrong type of tree for its setting, a tree brought from shores afar, affected by too much or too little water.

And with that in mind I refer you to a Pagan song of meaning by Mike Scott of The Waterboys, 'Church Not Made With Hands'.

On returning to Mahabalipuram, and after a few more days relaxing, the urge to move on came to the fore, so the four of us travelled north to Chennai with a connecting train up to the state of Odisha, where the main attractions were the temples of Bhubaneswar, the sun temple at Konark and the east coast seaside resort of Puri. And it was the latter that we made our base, for Puri is one of the holiest Hindu pilgrimage sites of India, famous for its annual Rath Yatra Festival where the idols of Lord Jagannath, Balbhadra and Subhadra are moved out of the Jagannath Temple, and whilst seated on chariots in ceremonial procession are drawn along the grand avenue by devotees to the Gundicha Temple some two miles away. Our time in Puri did not fall at such a busy time, and after negotiating a price in a lodge at the Western travellers' end of

THE DRUID IN THE GREENHOUSE

the beach, it provided for all our needs, including the hiring of bicycles, as we settled in for a relaxing and interesting stay. One has to be born into a Hindu family, and a sign at the Jagannath Temple states that non-Hindus are not allowed entry, apparently it goes back to the time of British rule. Being a holy place, Puri attracts Western devotees of Sri Krishna, and many can be seen and heard muttering mantras around the tight streets of the city.

The ancient World Heritage sun temple at Konark fired my imagination, but on enquiring there were only two buses a day from Puri, and as we wished to experience the sun temple at dusk, it would have to be an overnight stay.

My wife and I packed an overnight bag, took the morning bus, and on arrival at what appeared to be little more than a small one-street village, booked into the tourist bungalow directly opposite the temple gates. It was extremely hot, and with the bungalow having its own restaurant and with a couple of other places providing chai, snacks and cool drinks, there was little hardship to be had.

The bungalow had a number of rooms available but being midweek, the place was noticeably quiet, in fact apart from two male Vietnamese Buddhist practitioners, we were the only non-local folk around. After a wander and a light lunch followed by a siesta, the evening came around, with the strength of the sun declining the heat of the day still remained, and after an early meal we headed over the road to the great structure. The entrance saw us pass by the sentries of stone lions and elephants, our first impressions sailed high, it was the sheer magnitude of the building that rose up before us. Upon closer inspection the entire structure was that of a ginormous chariot of the sun god, Surya. The base of the chariot had a dozen wheels on either side and remained ready to be pulled by figures of horses; the mighty walls of the temple were covered in stone carvings, the seated figures of Surya the sun god, Chandra the goddess of the moon, Mars, Mercury, Jupiter, Venus, Saturn and along with Ketu and Rahu of the north and south nodes, confirmed the knowledge and the skills of its creators. With the sun going down the external lighting highlighted sections of the great mass of being, and on wandering around to check out the sound of voices, the shapes of the two Vietnamese men could be seen on a ledge high above. Upon descending the men informed us they were archaeologists visiting the ancient sites of this land, and as darkness overcame light, we made our way out of the site, and on stopping to reflect and stare skywards, felt humbled to sense, and witness the heavenly celestial dance. It is a strange thing that as children growing up, apart from a nursery rhyme involving a dish and a spoon, we were never taught anything about the sun and the moon. Upon rising the next morning, we ate the breakfast on offer, settled the bill, and stepped outside to board the bus back to Puri. It was a pleasant coastal journey, highlighted when a gentleman and his goat boarded the bus, and on taking a seat adjacent to ours, 'the little dog laughed to see so much fun' came to mind. After a few more days of comfortable living, we handed back the cycles, checked out of the lodge and took a rickshaw to the rail station, and on saying final goodbyes to our two friends, my wife and I took our seats for the start of an eight-hour northerly journey to Kolkata. However, it was not so straight forward as we had to change trains, and after five hours we disembarked onto a platform at Kharagpur Junction, and on doing so entered into a period of semi-madness.

The station was remarkably busy with a movement of multitudes of folk, and with trains arriving and departing all around us, we only had a short time to make our connection, the pressure was on. Public announcements filled the air but unfortunately meant nothing to us, and on asking non-English speaking platform attendants and porters they all gave different advice, and we ended up missing the connection. And so, it was time to take stock, and at such times it is best to purchase a drink just sit down and relax, and within the workings of India, a short time later an English-speaking, badge-wearing man appeared and in a statesman-like manner informed us that the Kolkata express train had just departed. And there wasn't another express train for hours; the remaining option was to board the commuter train that stood empty on the adjoining platform. On thanking the official, we hauled on our rucksacks and climbed into a carriage that had a startling effect, for apart from damage seats and dodgy-looking windows, the floors of the carriage were covered with rubbish: empty cups, newspapers, crushed boxes piled high in the aisles in a manner that resembled the morning after the finale act at a large outdoor music event. And with an acceptance of fate, we took two seats, and whilst sitting and staring the breeze of cold reality enhanced the scene, a young feral girl of around four or five years entered the carriage barefooted.

She was a sweet-looking thing in a raggedy mess, and with a small brush and a plastic bag in hand, crouched down on the floor and proceeded to syphon through the rubbish. We watched on as she selected her targets, placing anything seemingly semi-worthless inside her dirty dress, whilst plastic bottles went into the bag. She went about her work as if we were not there, and as the gap between us narrowed, a closer view revealed a set of sparkling eyes below matted hair no doubt infested with crawling head lice.

She was a dishevelled young soul whose very presence had an unsettling effect, being moved by her demeanour my wife made contact, and as she cautiously came closer, she revealed a smile of the sunflower, and like two scarecrows in a field of compassion, we slipped her some cash. It is hard for us to accept that she was the norm for a railway/street child, just one of so many 'untouchables' that are open to abuse whilst living a feral existence, and as the commuters piled into the carriage, she half turned, gave a fleeting smile, and disappeared into a sea of tailored shirts and saris. The train pulled out and picked up speed and all seemed good, that was until it began to stop and pick-up passengers every few minutes, and in a short time the carriage turned into a set from a movie. For if you can imagine a packed tube train in London, and then add loud and colourful women selling all manner of wares, and as they struggle to pass textile goods across your face and over your head, young girls proceed to sell bracelets and necklaces at chest level. And along with small boys offering sweets and nuts at waist height, in a sweaty carriage that lacked air conditioning, life at times can be grim. But it was the turning of a mind to amusement that provided the means to handle the day. In summary, you may hear it said that people from the West travel to India to find themselves, but what does that actually mean? It remains the norm that on the surface most people do not respond in that way, they may carry on from birth to death without giving it much thought, which is until a major incident happens and affects their lives. Whereas the person with the ambition to seek the truth is driven onwards by a strong desire to bring about inner change. As Westerners we are encouraged to do all sorts of things to strengthen and improve our bodies, and especially so when it involves outdoor activities which are beneficial and may well bring about mental relief. However, that only remains so up to a point, for if one is dedicated to training the mind, then the established practices of the East remain available, but be aware that the answer to the questions one seeks may well be hidden within a spiritual mine field.

On arrival at Kolkata's Howrah rail station, we held back to allow fellow rushing commuters space to disembark, and on looking down at the remains on the carriage floor, it all starts again. On fixing our rucksacks and stepping out we strode past platform porters in red waistcoats with huge moustaches and on leaving the station behind, entered into a mass insect-like setting. And after somehow negotiating a price with a taxi wallah, we climbed into his Ambassador car and joined the queue to cross over the giant Meccano set that is Howrah

Bridge. For a foreign person travelling to India for the first time, Kolkata would not be a choice of destination, for it is as far removed from a popular resort like Goa, a comparison to a drink-fuelled hen party attempting to cross Helvellyns striding edge in bad weather. For on crossing the Hooghly River, an arm of the sacred Ganga, one could not help but notice the hardships that the residents of this great city must constantly endure. We hadn't pre-booked a place to stay, but on referring to the now battered *Lonely Planet*, we informed the driver to take us to the Chowringhee district's Sudder Street area, a place geared up for foreign tourists. And having lived modestly for the past few weeks we had budgeted for a more upmarket place to stay, and with a little persuasion managed to book ourselves into a double room at the Lytton Hotel.

The area provided plenty of places to eat, drink and chill, but it was the soul of the streets, observing the families who live out openly on the pavements, the ones you step over on your return journey each night. And along with the human-powered rickshaw pullers who run barefooted with hand bells and sweat soaked rags, it is the ugliness of sheer beauty that strikes the gong of empathy. Visiting the Maidens where cricket is played, the avenues of grand colonial houses and the large Victorian buildings where we were ushered aside to allow police officers to whack the gathering locals with sticks of cane. The markets and botanical gardens where monkeys did play, the bustle and packed dilapidated trams that passed churches, temples, mosques, and the YMCA. For although squalor and riches lay side by side, it is the naked humour and the beauty of the people of place that illuminates one's soul. And having said that we both got ill, my wife at first, caught a bug of the stomach that meant weakness and starvation for at least a few days, however hers cleared up, but I was less fortunate. The plan was to head north to Darjeeling, see the tea-picking ladies, visit a couple of Tibetan monasteries, ride on the toy train, and simply soak in the beauty that the land has to offer. After an early rise and a taxi ride to Kolkata's Sealdah rail station, we arrived to find a colourful setting of awaiting passengers rising from slumber. We found our seats on the train to New Jalpaiguri, and for the first time during the trip there were a good number of other Westerners who had boarded the train, and the setting for the four-plus-hour journey had an atmosphere of joy. Twangs of Aussies and Kiwis mixed in with the banter of Germans, Swiss, Brits and Danes could be heard above the motion of the rattling train, and as it squeezed itself around the Bangladesh border, the mighty Ganges River flowed with the life and soul of the region.

On arrival at our destination, it got a bit confusing as New Jalpaiguri and Silguri both have rail stations but appear to be one and the same place, for those northern readers a bit like the cities of Manchester and Salford. However, with a little further research I learnt that the Silguri line went north whilst the New Jalpaiguri Junction ran east to west. And on leaving the station the choices to get to Darjeeling were laid out before us: we could get a bus, wait for the toy train that took hours or jump into a shared jeep. And with the latter being the main form of transport around the region, we teamed up with like-minded travellers and on squeezing into the vehicles headed north in a convey of anticipation. Climbing higher and higher past small villages with waiting Sherpas that relied on the toy train, we stopped for a quick snack at a village location, where a local man offered a view of a piece of a yeti for a small price. Back on board we passed a large monastery before arriving at our destination, the Hill Cart Road station. The town of Darjeeling straddles a ridge at 2,134 metres above sea level and provides plenty of scope to get fit, and with rucksacks getting heavier we headed on up towards the traveller's area around the TV tower. After a gruelling twenty-minute walk we arrived at the top of the ridge, then stuck to a well-rehearsed plan. My wife would stay with the bags whilst I would set off looking for a suitable place to stay, and in line with the workings of life, it could happen in an instant or take up a good part of the day. With an eye on the budget, we booked in for a week's stay in a popular backpacker's place, run by a Sherpa family, whose members all oozed friendliness. We settled into a room upstairs at the back, the walls and ceilings were covered with timber panelling and it had a good feel, but on viewing from the outside, the room was actually suspended out across the ridge on wooden stilts. And with a major drop below us we had to accept that if the structure gave way during our stay, then so be it.

As night-time came rats could clearly be heard living and moving around in the voids behind the room's wooden panelling, but after a quick check there were no passages of entry, we placed our thoughts into the box of acceptance. But that was not my only concern, as my stomach pains that started on the train were worsening, my physical health was deteriorating at a fast rate. With lower cramps and a constant stream of foul liquid, I stopped eating for a couple of days, but that had little effect, so I made my way to the local clinic.

I was impressed when almost immediately I received service, and on handing over a few rupees I was informed that I had dysentery, but in order to prescribe the correct medication I would be required to provide a test sample.

But a problem arose when I was informed that it was festival time and the laboratory was closed, so I would have to wait three more days for the test results. And during that period, I got worse, much worse, and so I took to carrying around the three sacred objects, one of water, a toilet roll, and a pack of incense sticks. Whilst having to constantly drink water to prevent dehydration, and with violent stomach cramps kicking like a hare trapped in a sack, I never strayed too far from home. After a torrid few days, I returned to the clinic to be met by a friendly and knowledgeable female doctor who herself had worked in the UK, and after a few more tests prescribed me with the correct medication to treat my symptoms. And within three days I had made a rapid improvement, and yes, I had lost a few stone, but I was pleased that my spirits had remained good throughout the experience. After a walk in some woodland and much to the appreciation of a group of local young lads I ended up joining in a game of cricket, a game that became a series between India and England in the first test at Darjeeling.

I had no idea who won, for I ended up playing for both sides, and when the homemade stumps were lifted, the locals came together to cheer us on our way. Darjeeling, the Queen of the Himalayas, on a cloudless day can offer stunning and breathtaking views, and during our stay we were rewarded with a glimpse of the world's third highest mountain, Kanchenjunga. The area had plenty of things on offer, from a journey on the amazing toy train, a visit to the fabulously located and famous Yogachoeling Gompa, with a splash-out coming in the form of afternoon tea at the Observatory Hill's colonial Windamere Hotel. At times when travelling around visiting places and taking in the sights and sounds, I find little time for personal practice, for it is more about absorbing the moment. But I do recall an early morning wander along the ridge, the town was still in the process of awaking, and with few folk about, I managed to spend some time alone in contemplation. Sat high at a lovely spot, sharing space amongst the trees I managed to slip away, and as prayer flags moved in gentle motion with the feel of the coming breeze, the smile of the universe stroked my soul. On travels I judge a place by asking myself if I could live there permanently, and the answer for Darjeeling was yes, we both could. After a hearty breakfast and a good cup of Yorkshire-like tea, we said our goodbyes to Darjeeling, paid for two seats in a shared jeep, and whilst sat tight amongst a friendly Ghurkha family, set off in an eastly direction. And as the bare thread tyres of the jeep trundled along the road passing the plantations where ladies at work picked tea, we arrived in good time at Kalimpong, our next place of stay.

The driver dropped us off at the main bus stand, and after a good stretch, we carried our bags a few paces before taking some seats outside a local café, and with coffees and pastries on order, we took time to take stock. Once revitalised, and with clear bearings, we went round the corner and booked into a cheap and friendly lodge, and it was a pleasant surprise to find our tidy first-floor room overlooked the courtyard of the local mosque, and with a window in line with the minaret, it provided a pleasant change. For having spent a decade working and living amongst Muslim people, I had gained some knowledge of the Five Pillars of Islam and having only recently lived within ear shot of mosques in the Gulf, we decided to leave the window open. And it was sometime later and during the hours of darkness, when I was alerted by the familiar sound of a tap on a microphone, and with the moon of the night casting its shadow came the enchanting sound of the muezzin as he called his congregation to prayer. It was the sheer beauty of the area that had brought us to Kalimpong, a small town straddled across a ridge in the foothills and being lower than Darjeeling offered clearer views.

After breakfast and a nosey around town, we set off walking up a steep hill to visit the Tibetan Tharpa Choling Gompa, the home of the Yellow Hats. But on arrival we discovered that the place did not feel right, although some monks were in attendance, it felt flat and devoid of energy. Although disappointing the setting and the views all around made it worthwhile and having noticed a nice spot we sat down to eat our packed lunch. But it wasn't long, maybe only a minute, before we got into conversation with a local man, who I noticed was wearing an old-style Chelsea FC shirt below his jacket. As it turned out, he used to live and work in west London, and had been a regular season ticket holder at Stamford Bridge. After declaring his passion for the club and his memories of being in the shed end, I provided him with a catch-up, as best as I could. On explaining why we were sat on the ground near his home, he informed us that the Gompa had fallen into disarray when the head Lama and some senior monks had gone off to America. On hearing those words, and with tongue in cheek, I couldn't help but ask if they had gone to Disneyland. He shared the joke, but informed us that it was all really sad, as they were hearing strong rumours that they were never to return. The Gompa was now more or less shut down, the remaining monks had lost their direction, and in fact one or two had become depressed. He went on to inform us that for safe keeping, all the religious artefacts brought over the mountains from Lhasa had been removed from the Gompa and taken to a place further up the ridge. And with a glint in his eye, he asked if we would like to see them. Well, my immediate thought was one of caution, but on quizzing him further, he informed us that having been raised in a house opposite the Gompa, he had grown up knowing all the monks. Although he was a Hindu, similar to me he held a fascination for Tibet, their beliefs, and practices, and having declared he had no desire for payment, he turned and disappeared into the Gompa. In a short time he returned holding a large rusty key, and it was with a sense of magic that we strode up the steep hill, and as each boot heel came down on the ground, we became part of the panoramic view. Our West End guide came into his own as he pointed and named the high peaks, the valleys, the distant villages, and the landmarks in his township below. On arrival at the old building, excitement filled the air, our guide led us down a bank, before we came to a halt at a solid looking door.

On inserting and turning the key, he slowly pushed it open, and as we entered a large darkish room, it was with a sense of wonder that I can only describe the experience, as being one similar to that of entry into the main chamber of an Egyptian tomb. For as our eyes adjusted with the shimmering light from the open door, statues, and numerous figures of the Tibetan Gelug sect, the one of His Holiness the Dalai Lama appeared before us. As we stood in awe, our newfound friend who by now was overcome with joy began to remove the layers of dusty cloth sheets and sacking. And in doing revealed deities, and Dharma protectors, golden artefacts, and a figure I recognised, that of Je Tsongkhapa, the founder of the tradition. These were figures you would normally see on display in cabinets and behind sheets of glass in main monasteries. A further scan of the room revealed piles of Tibetan framed paintings, whilst thangkas and mandalas could be seen stacked up tight against crumbling walls. And like supervised children inside a toy shop we were given permission to explore, yet it didn't feel right just to rummage, so we moved around the room with respect, and on climbing around some closed trunks, the lids were raised to reveal parchments, and collections of smaller ceremonial items, bells, and handheld musical instruments, bronze vajras and plates with distinguished markings. And on the lifting of sheets in the corner, we were amazed by the sight of a line of huge ceremonial horns, a sight that instantly brought back images of the old film footage of 1950s Lhasa. But sadly, just like the Gompa down the hill, the storehouse held a lost feel, the artefacts had gone flat, but it left me with a feeling that it only needed a ceremony with the use of the large horns, and the place would become re-energised and the spirit would return. Similar to a line of steam locomotives standing motionless and soulless inside an old engine shed. Then as soon as the fireman arrives and sets to work with the four elements, the fire, and the power of steam, brings them back to life once more. But our spirits remained high as we walked back down the hill, the key was returned to the Gompa, and as the Chelsea fan had an errand to do, he accompanied us back down the hill into town, on arrival at the post office shop, we said our goodbyes. The whole experience left me with a strange feeling of misplacement, a sort of going to see a play at a theatre to find the wrong props for the setting. During my life whenever I see or have visited strange or isolated settings, I may spend time wondering what sort of a person I would have become if I had been raised there? And this was one of those occasions. Prior to leaving Darjeeling and in tune with other Westerners, we had spent a few hours visiting various official buildings to obtain paperwork and visas to enter the northern state of Sikkim, a small strip of land squeezed in between Nepal, Bhutan, and Tibet. And after settling our bill and saying our goodbyes at the guest house, we jumped into a shared jeep, and set off on a five-hour journey into Sikkim, and its capital Gangtok. Apart from the wonder of the landscape one of the interesting experiences of the pleasant journey was the Sikkim border town of Rangpo, a place where almost every shop and business appeared to be involved in the distribution and sale of alcohol, a sort of Himalayan version of a Calais alcohol superstore.

Our stay in Gangtok was memorable. It was a Saturday morning, my wife was having her hair cut, and after a while of wandering around I returned to the salon to be offered a seat and a drink. So, I sat there observing Tibetan ladies having their hair braided and styled with head ornaments containing fabric material, strings of corals, turquoises, and mosaics in line with their tradition. We stayed in a travellers' lodge run by two brothers, who arranged a social day out. It was a journey in shared jeeps up towards the Tibetan border, where after a walk up to the top of a snow-covered ridge we came down to be met by colourful ladies in traditional garments who provided warm drinks from corrugated shacks, and on being surrounded by prayer flags we took pictures of chilled-out yaks. We found Gangtok to be a friendly place, like the time in a café, a monk with a can of Coca-Cola in hand came over and asked if he could join us for a chat. It was where we were first introduced to the huge Tibetan mastiffs, but it was the Tsang Apsos that stole our hearts, especially the one sat outside our lodgings who needed a bath. And after a week of walking and strolling around, visiting the sites and sampling local delicacies, it was time to book a shared jeep. The start of a journey that would take us back down to New Jalpaiguri Junction, and a sleeper train to the Mughalsarai, a station lying just 8 miles south of the ancient city of Varanasi.

THE DRUID IN THE GREENHOUSE

'Enter the light of the dawn of day and be seated in unity at the table of peace.'
Des

BRIDGES AND FUNERAL PYRES

As the old saying goes the pleasure is in getting there, and for me the overnight train journey, like all journeys across India can deliver fascinating experiences. Around 2 am with most passengers asleep, the train slowly made its way through Bihar, the birthplace of the Buddha, yet considered the unruliest of states. I could be observed taking banter with two-night stewards in the next compartment, and like the motion of a giant python we slid into the capital's station that is Patna. The stewards informed me we were due for a lengthy stop, and as the doors of the carriage opened, I stepped out into the dimly lit station.

The place had a presence, for it came with an aura of red and a distinct feel of the medieval. The air was sticky, spindly porters of the night unloaded parcels, faces constantly wiped with sweat rags, then placed over shoulders in a manner of correct dress. Even the pigeons seemed affected. In fact, with a deeper intake of breath, you could taste the effects of pollution.

I crossed the platform and took a seat on an empty goods trolley, relaxed, aware of absorbing the feel of place. Further down the eerie platform and within earshot I observed a group of about twenty or so military-like ruffians, armed with old rifles, an image of an old Mexican western movie came to mind. Straddled in a somewhat loose manner, before them stood a leader who pointed and shouted out orders. Suddenly they all turned and set off down the platform searching, and as they sought and probed alongside the standing carriages of our train, I consciously slipped into a cloak of invisibility.

Two passed right beside me without even a glance, but then a thought occurred, what if I were to be arrested and taken away, my wife would wake up in the morning to discover that I had vanished, disappeared in the night, how would she feel and what would she do? And with that thought in mind I slipped back into the carriage unnoticed. Life looked sweet for the two black swans who had made their home on the lily-covered lake, for it was still just about dark when the train pulled into Mughalsarai Junction.

On leaving the station we were greeted by the usual crowd of men, a sea of now familiar faces, all offering various modes of transport to our given destinations. We discussed our options, and having been offered an alternative quicker route, we agreed a fare with an enthusiastic driver, climbed into the back of his motorised rickshaw, and set off on the final leg of our journey to the holy city of Varanasi. 'This quick way, quick way,' repeated the driver. y now cockerels could be heard announcing the arrival of a brand-new day, villages were awakening, figures of those who chose to sleep outside could be seen rising from charpoy beds. And as we rumbled on with the first rays of the sun of the day casting its light, ablution time, locals could

THE DRUID IN THE GREENHOUSE

be seen with tin and towel in hand, slowly making their way towards the surrounding fields where earlier arrivals bobbed up and down beside buffalo and egret. At roadside standpipes, folk could be observed collecting water for their masala chai boilers, others simply stood and washed, clearing, and swilling their throats, a sound and scene since time immemorial. It was a special dawn breaking, as our spirited driver repeated his personal shortcut mantra and through the rising morning mist, we caught site of a floating pontoon bridge. And as our little vehicle mounted the wooden boards of the floating structure, like the wingspan of a wandering albatross, the whole width of the mighty Ganges lay before us.

As the feel of coldness rose up from the water, the enormity of the task ahead came home, our little rickshaw bobbed and swayed to the pulling power as we advanced slowly along planks of a once temporary floating bridge. It was at this point of realisation, that no sane Westerner would ever do anything like this in their own place of abode; however, here it was the norm. It was still very early, and the bridge was empty, and my quick risk assessment revealed that if today was to be our last, then drowning in the mighty Ganges was our destiny, and so embrace it, we did.

About halfway across, the pontoon bowed to the pull of the strong current, and with water splashing over the top of our tiny tin covered scooter, our driver laughed loudly as he struggled to keep us on track. And like a clockwork mouse navigating its way across a living room floor on Christmas morning, everything became as one, the now embracing action of the rickshaw took us ever closer to the far bank, and with a motion akin to the turning of a pop-up page, an unbelievable sight came into view. Conceptual rhubarb and custard, the dawning of Varanasi, standing alive and majestic, its feet grounded within an evocative mist that rose like a water dragon from the holy waters of Mother Ganga. A sacred icon seen shimmering beneath the golden breath of divine grace. And as the bow in the pontoon eased, we began to accelerate, and with a straight line laid out before us, it came with a sense of relief, when our little mouse landed and sped away onto firmer ground. Within the scale of the boiling of two kettles, we were dropped off outside our pre-booked Shivala Ghat guest house, paid, and waved our goodbyes to the trusted driver, who with a final exuberant cry sped away down the dusty street. After a decent breakfast on the rooftop terrace, we placed our rucksacks inside our sparse prison-cell-like room, and with the city now awakened it was time to step out and explore.

Varanasi an ancient city, one of the holiest pilgrim destinations in India, famous for its numerous ghats where Hindus come to bathe in the sacred waters of the Ganges. A place where near-naked ascetics, followers of Shiva with matted hair and faces covered with spent ash from funeral pyres, sit absorbing hot charas from tapered chillums.

It is the 'burning ghats' the places of open cremations that provide the star attraction for the Western traveller, a unique location, where timber-loaded boats offload their cargo onto its rising steps.

A place where the senses go into overdrive, making way

as the carriers of the dead slip by, and with the sights of multiple cremations, comes the smells of burning incense, and the taste of death itself. A scene overlaid with the sound of the rites, the chanting of sacred hymns, and as the flames of the fire dies down, the cracking of sculls, whilst remains are gathered by those untouched, then slipped away into the sacred waters of Mother Ganga. Westerners may well arrive at the burning ghats with a fear, a preconceived view of a daily show, a live act of life and death played out on a giant stage set before peering eyes. Intrigued by how many older Hindu folk make a life-planned long pilgrimage to this holy city simply to await death can be a bit full on for the unexposed Western mind. During our stay we shared conversation with a mature woman who had moved to the city three years earlier. She had expected to die within a short period of arrival, but she recovered, and bizarrely became trapped. For she feared that if she returned home, or even left Varanasi for a day she may die, and all her efforts would have been in vain. And as heavy swans run across water to take flight, so too is the acceptance of the cycle of life and death, and the belief that on entering the spiritual purifying waters of the Ganga, the reincarnation cycle will end, and they will reach nirvana. The mid-morning air was strong with the smells of Indian street life, and after a drink and a snack and without a need to hurry, we slowly made our way to an area where access to the waterfront could only be obtained through a series of small alleyways. Whilst peacefully strolling down a passageway, shielded from light by tall buildings, the scene suddenly changed. A shout, followed by the sound of hooves clunking on well-worn flag stones, we had to react, tucking up tight against the smeared walls of time, when a line of enthusiastic water-buffalo emerged on their way down to the river. Once again it was as though we were not there, the spanning horns of beasts raised some alarm, their bodies brushed against ours, we could smell their odour, large dark eyes, bulging nostrils played tunes with the tightness of the air, as the beautiful creatures breezed by. They were on a mission, driven on by familiarity and the smell of water, whilst we just hoped that our feet would be spared from the motion of heavy hooves. And with the sight of the last tail disappearing around a narrow corner, the experience ended when a stooped muttering man, with small stick, passed by.

It is a funny thing that in India the visitor can be the centre of attraction or just an invisible soul, the latter being the case this time. The buffalo had been kind to us. However, a few months early whilst walking to a bank on a busy road, a passing sacred cow decided to butt me in the right thigh; it was only a turn of the neck to let me know who was in charge, but I certainly knew about it. Time spent wandering the streets and rear squares of the city gave rise to new experiences, one began where we came across a large gathering of men, and on investigation it turned out to be a court followed by an orderly public beating. A senior man who appeared to be in charge came over and offered a silly explanation for the gathering, and on realising that we were not buying his story, went on to explain that the man was a thief, and the punishment was being delivered by his victim. It is good to remember that when travelling around the planet, and especially in countries like India, it is wise to adapt a policy that we are just there to observe, to sample, to move on without judgement. Law and order must have been on the menu for us in Varanasi, for the following night whilst reading inside our cell, I heard a commotion outside. On rising and staring through the barred window, I witnessed a large group of men carrying burning torches leading three roped men down the street, I left that one to the imagination. After a few more nights' stay in the city, we decided we needed to chill, and relocated to the Cantonment area.

On the cab journey out from the old city there is an intriguing place, and one well worth a mention; it is a location where all roads converge to meet as one below a bridge, but there is nothing attached to the bridge, just an old structure standing alone below a network of overhead cables. But the area is full of people on the move, and on final approaches the over-laden trucks, taxis, rickshaws, family members sharing scooters, wandering sacred cows, ladies carrying pots on their heads, porters with huge packs on their backs, all enthusiastically headed towards the bridge.

With the sounds of the traffic, the bells and the horns and the shouting of men, like participants in a snail race we crawled into line and became squashed into the bottle neck below the lone structure. For us with no real rush to get anywhere, the passage through the bridge became a highlight. On another occasion we passed through beside a group of monkey people, devotees of the god Hanuman, dressed in half ape clothing and with faces painted could be seen carrying lines of cable complete with bulbs above their heads. At the rear of an old flat back truck, cables met, a seated man on a bicycle beside batteries used pedal power to operate the lighting set-up. And with an intake of breath, we all squeezed through. I asked our driver why they did not just remove the bridge, he looked at me as being plain stupid, and repeated, 'Bridge very old.'

His answer brought back memories of a previous conversation I had with a taxi driver, I cannot recall the place, only that it was in central India. Whilst sat in a rickshaw approaching a roundabout in traffic, I noticed a man on a moped. What made him stand out was his pillion passenger, the figure of a large monkey seated upright with its arms wrapped around his waist. On noting that down in the book of most intriguing, I left it at that, but a couple of days later when attempting to cross a road in dense traffic, I caught another glimpse of the fleeting twosome. Towards the end of the week when visiting an area for reasons long forgotten, a large gang of mischievous monkeys could be seen and heard scampering around on rooftops. The macaques usually hang around places where easy pickings can be had, sometimes entering residential districts getting what they can before moving on. Occasionally, as in this case, they chose to stay, to steal, cause damage and create general havoc. Watching the commotion with a mind of comedy and intrigue, I asked an observing taxi driver what was going on. He informed me that he lived locally, and the macaques had been around for days; the residents had had enough so they called for the monkey man. India is a place that appears crazy, yet it actually works, and this piece of information confirmed that fact. It now made sense, for the man on the moped and his langur were actually partners in business. On receiving a call, they rode into the residential area, the langur leapt off the bike, and with a high-pitched screaming sound, sent the smaller macaque running for fear of their lives. Job done the macaques moved on, the monkey man got paid. After watching the show, I questioned the taxi driver as to why the locals just didn't play a recorded sound of the langur? The answer: 'The man and his monkey would have no work.' However, a few years later I learnt that the Delhi authorities had banned the use of langurs, and now employ men to mimic its sound, but upon hearing that news, I felt saddened.

Travelling around and especially when staying in places like Varanasi, the way of life can be somewhat basic, for after living in cells with squats, and red lights to keep the down the mosquitoes, every now and again it was refreshing to splash out, spend a few nights in a manner more in keeping with a Western lifestyle. The Cantonment area has most of the cities more upmarket accommodation and we found a place with a well-kept lawn garden, that also allowed large motor homes to park up. The Surya Hotel, named after the Hindu god of the sun, had a main building, but we chose to stay in the single floor chalet-like rooms located around the lawn. With a veranda and air conditioning and being isolated from the smells and sounds of the bustling city, it was a good place to chill, recharge batteries, simply take stock. After fully unpacking for the first time in a long while, finding things that had been lost forever,

THE DRUID IN THE GREENHOUSE

I decided to take a seat on the veranda and enjoy the flora and fauna of the well-kept gardens. But in sync with life in general and especially when travelling, there is always a twist, and it is wise to remain aware and be prepared for the unexpected. During the travels I continued to study Hindu spiritual teachings. It was the second day of our stay when I became aware of activity in the larger room next door. A conference was in motion. Now at home in the West this could have had negative repercussions, with a potential for the rise of anxiety, resulting in anger. But with an Indian-like mindset, the best choice is to wait and see the outcome, to look for the positives that may at first be hidden before judgement is made. Being pre-monsoon season, it was hot and sticky so the conference room doors were left open, and whilst sitting out on the veranda the strong clear voice of an Indian man could be heard addressing the room, to my delight a guru delivering yogic teachings to a group of English-speaking students. I could clearly hear every word spoken, and fortunately I had some understanding as to the context of his presentation, and it laid down the roots for an enjoyable stay, especially after meeting the friendly guru at lunchtime, who after a long chat invited me to join in his lessons free of charge. But somehow that didn't feel right, so I opted instead to adjust my seating to a place out on the veranda in front of the conference room. One evening we did venture out to a neighbouring upmarket hotel, where on arrival we were greeted by exuberant staff wearing fine traditional costume. Led away into luxurious surroundings, beautiful gardens with outdoor pool, a restaurant with bar serving pricy exotic cocktails, delivered to the background sound of a classical Indian raga. It was all very nice and thoroughly enjoyable, but for me on such occasions, as it still does to this day, holds an underlying feeling of unease, for the delivery of extravagance being played out before us, as the poor hotel and restaurant staff and family musicians looked on, not to mention the untouchables, those souls raking and clearing the funeral pyres down at the ghats.

There is a saying 'Man cannot see because he has eyes'

And whilst staying in Varanasi we took the opportunity to have a day out: Sarnath, the place where upon achieving enlightenment the Buddha first taught the Dharma, delivered his 'Sermon in the Deer Park' setting out the doctrines of the Four Noble Truths. Sarnath is also famous for its third-century stupa, erected by the emperor Ashoka and the famous lion-capital memorial pillar, which is now the state emblem of India. It may also be worthy of note that the centre of the Indian Flag bears the Dharma wheel or Ashoka Chakra, the wheel of duty with its 24 spokes, religious paths made for humans. A site of distinction with numerous Mahayana and Theravadin temples and shines representing Buddhism from different lands. Like a trolley run in a supermarket, it was a Jain temple that guided us down its aisle, for on entry it oozed pure serenity, as its gentle cupped hands had a cradling effect upon the soul. I first became aware of Jains in the 1960s, and had looked in on them along the way, picking shreds of knowledge, their beliefs, and practices, especially those of protecting miniscule creatures. Having eaten out at Jain restaurants where onions and garlic are proscribed, this menu had much more to offer. So, we took the opportunity to simply sit down in peace, to contemplate, to meditate and become one in a setting of bliss. But after a while the arrival of a group of very loud and enthusiastic Indian male tourists sounded the signal that our time was up, returning once more into the fold that is samsara, the binding realm of material existence. Back at the hotel and after a final lunch we were grateful to have sampled a few days of luxury and learning. It was with a touch of loss that we snaked our way through the noble bridge, onwards towards the railway station, where two pre-booked seats on the 28-hour Ratnagiri Express overnight sleeper train to Mumbai awaited. And as the train slowly made its way across the huge steel bridge that spans the mighty Ganges, a spot where locals fish from boats with magnets, attempting to catch coins thrown as final offerings from train windows. Unusually for me, a backwards glance towards the burning ghats of Varanasi. With that last glance came a knowing, as I left for the final time, like their fathers before them, the young funeral pyre builders will themselves grow old and die. And as the cities ancient name changes from Kashi to Benares and now Varanasi, the way will simply go on, just as it has, throughout recorded time. The train picked up speed, Ravi Shankar played Kathakali Kathak, and as we settled in for a long journey, it was a time to reflect on those gifts received during our stay in the ancient city of Shiva. For as a Westerner, words of decay and death are seldom spoken. In fact, we mistakenly see death as darkness, not as a passage of light. We assume a linear life where everything is laid out in turn, with a standpoint where life should end when we are old, although the age is not forthcoming. And when a person unfortunately dies before three score years and ten, we say they went early, as that was no age at all. Yet, people die young and especially when in tragic circumstances one may question the existence of God, and how can he be so cruel, and you may hear it said that God works in mysterious ways. Whilst sat back at home in a cosy armchair, I recently watched a travel programme where the likeable presenter Simon Reeve visited the burning ghats of Varanasi. And whilst there he became visibly affected by the in-your-face experience, and the ease in which the Hindu people accept death. Raised within a Western capitalist system, we are encouraged to go for it, to obtain material goods and to live the dream. But in doing we develop a strong sense of self- importance, an attachment to objects gained, with a developing fear of losing them. In India one of the ever occurring and noticeable sites is that of the immaculately dressed school children, who each day excitedly leave their humble dwellings and head off to school. On arrival they form a sea of happy smiling faces that simply radiate life, and those little bobbing boats remain a shining example to us all. There is a saying 'Man cannot hear because he has ears' and here in the West, we remain ignorant, for being untrained we allow our self-grasping minds to bring forth discrimination, anger and hurt, not to mention the seeking out of our personal desires, those negative practices that have an effect on our emotions, and lead to suffering. Whereas the Dharma of the Indian people is to train and cultivate the mind, and in doing develop an understanding and a knowing that we are not the body, nor the intellect, and that only the physical body will decompose.

After our final overnight train journey, we experienced a delightful weeklong stay in the vibrant city of Mumbai, a place that comes into its own as darkness falls. It was late afternoon when we left our mid-range hotel, strolling at ease along wide tree-lined streets made up of lovely old colonial residential buildings, and as we moved closer to the seafront, we found a place to dine in nice settings. After paying our bill and a walk to Chowpatty beach, we set off back to our hotel, but as darkness descended the return revealed a different picture, for the once pleasant streets became home to hundreds of people.

Whole families frantically going about the task of making temporary night shelters out on pavements, and against the upright walls. Women could be seen cooking on stoves and open fires, children stayed close to mothers' hand, as men prepared concoctions to inject in their arms. Further along unaccountable amounts of people of all ages slept out on empty market stalls, rickshaw wallahs tucked up on back seats, and as the cities winged mammals replaced roosting starlings, we slipped by unnoticed.

The back wheels lifted, the aircraft ascended, it was goodbye India. Will she ever welcome my return?

ALBION RETURN

We needed to re-adjust, and after seven days visiting people and places in Qatar, we returned to the UK. Arriving at Heathrow jobless with nowhere to live, well chilled, and still in the travelling mode, we boarded a train and headed to Somerset, and the delightful city of Bath.

Back in the bungalow in Kerala it had come to me that for the next chapter of this life, I needed to discover more of my homeland, whilst learning and gaining experience as a speaker. In order to achieve a realistic goal, if your request has heart, we can ask the powers of the universe for guidance and support. And whilst the magic boomerang travels out through the galaxy, with a conscious knowing of one's destiny, we set out our stall in preparation for its return. We had been asked by a number of people why Bath? and our answer was we just liked it, and from a spiritual path perspective, it was where we were supposed to be. Having spent a few days visiting letting agencies we agreed to take up residence in a first-floor Georgian flat in Great Pulteney Street.

A central location, a motion to sample the delights of the city, with an ease to visit the ancient sites of the West Country.

Having spent months walking around the sites, valleys, and

mountains of India, I was delighted to discover just how hilly and quirky Bath actually was. And with the added bonus of a canal and two parks right on our doorstep, with a river within close proximity, it provided ample choices for outdoor sessions.

On Friday evenings we attended the local tai chi class, and like the gripping tail action of a kinkajou, life appeared relatively sweet.

Having returned from travelling with books of interest I took to in-depth studying of Indian philosophy, with the teachings of gurus, the Upanishads, and the practice of Vipassana Meditation. Living in Somerset proved to be both stimulating and rewarding, for apart from the facilities of nearby Bristol, the Mendips, and the beauty of the Levels, Wiltshire, and the coasts and moorlands of Devon and Cornwall were all within striking distance. And with the New Age scene evolving all around us, the word 'boredom' was seldom whispered. But as the round of life continued and normality returned, we both took jobs to support our savings. For me it was Bristol where I met and got to know younger work colleagues; I could see that the city was going through a stage of awakening, new seeds being sown, nutrients added, and on more recent returns, the fruits of the harvest are there to see. After a year in Bath, with daughter having returned from the Gulf, and mainly due to aging parents requiring some support, we took the decision to return back north. Some may say 'It's grim up north', and that's one state of mind, but on observing clean washing blowing on a line in the front garden of a Yorkshire High Street house, that's another.

But as expected, it was not easy, yet after a couple of topsy-turvy years, things started to fall in place. We all had incomes, got back into hill walking, and had the pleasures of a new puppy dog. And for me, a new industry, one that provided the means to travel around the UK and across to Ireland, and with the added bonus of also becoming a trainer, the boomerang had returned to hand. And so, with the path of the seeker once more at the forefront, my task was to remove those hidden barriers, and in some cases pull down barricades and the force fields of resistance. Upon reflection of this lifetime, I had gained some knowledge, drawn from a collection of belief systems ranging from the Testaments of the Bible, Christianity, Colonel Gaddafi's Green Book to Native North and South American Indian, Hindu, Buddhist, Jain, Islamic and Taoist traditions, and throughout this period I had been a student of various forms of martial arts. And with the daily practice of meditation, tai chi and breathing techniques, I held a deep feeling for our planet and the whole of creation. A realisation that having reached a point on the journey, I had knowingly gathered together a full rucksack, a collection of non-joined-up spiritual experiences, not to mention its trivia. Being a solo seeker, driven on by a deep-rooted determination to arrive at a place I did not yet know, I needed to take stock. Throughout my life I had always had a liking to take on new challenges, whether it be spiritual, pastime activities or career based, and after having settled back down in the north, I made the decision to become self-employed. And in that motion, the refurbished lock gates began to ease open, and as new waters rushed in, it provided a way to greater freedom, with scope to ascend.

DEEP WORDS AND THE YEW SCHOOL TEACHERS

The birds around the car park garden were actively selecting the materials that form their unique nests. My task was to conduct a fire safety inspection of the care home. A couple of hours later inside a secure dementia wing, whilst concentrating on the job in hand, I heard a commotion, a sound of distress that appeared to be coming from a room further down the corridor.

Suddenly after a loud single shout, a tall figure of a man came running out of a bedroom, a nurse and carer followed in close pursuit. My attention switched to the man, who with his back to me was wearing only a vest and a nappy, he was crying out with words of no meaning. As staff members drew closer, he managed to remove and deposit his soiled nappy onto the corridor floor. A nurse caught up, and with kind words wrapped a towel around his waist. As they led him back towards his room, I looked into his deep-set eyes, a disturbing experience that exposed anguish and the helplessness of a man truly suffering. He was of a similar age to me, and in good physical shape, but the cold reality of the other side of life struck well and truly home. I was taken aback, touched, and with words spoken unintentionally, I stated

'I don't want to end up like that.'

Instantaneously a strong and powerful masculine voice, one that came from within and without replied, 'Then become a Celtic Shaman.'

'What?!' came my startled reply.

In a state of shock, I remained half-aware of the poor man being led away to his room, the bedroom door closed, and all in the corridor become still once more. The experience had clearly had an effect on me, and I was glad to finish the job and return to the car.

On the journey home, and with time to reflect, I understood that I was actually supposed to be there at that exact moment in time to witness the man's suffering. The following days after the care home experience were ones that involved deeper reflection and contemplation, the words of the voice had been delivered with a one-off firmness, a correction of pathway instruction. It was now down to me, my choice, and the way I responded would direct me on a course for the rest of this lifetime, the universe had spoken, and I accepted its advice. Laying aside all the experiences and the ups and downs of a life caused by my own actions, I had a core value, one with an inner directive, driven on by an end-goal determination. As a younger man and again in more recent times, I had been enthralled by a shamanic book, *The Teachings of Don Juan* by Carlos Castaneda, a man who had taken his readers into the world of Yaqui Indian sorcery. Having gained some knowledge of Tibetan Oracles, and those of distant lands, inspired I bought a book called *The Celtic Shaman* by the author John Mathews, a man distinguished in that field. I found the book interesting, and it motivated me to spend more time seeking further knowledge. It turned out that I didn't pursue it directly. However, the seeds had been sown, and on following my instinct, it was not very long before I landed at the door of Wicca. Back in the decades of time, I had been influenced by the myths and legends of Avalon, and like others had taken an interest in the ancient places of Albion, the circles of stones, the barrows, the ley lines and the beliefs and practices of the ancient ones, our ancestors. At the time I didn't really know anyone that I could discuss or seriously practise with, but it wasn't long before I followed the ways of the Pagan, albeit in the hedge, one might say.

My new occupation took me within striking distance of lots of way-out places, those historic and mystical sites that had stories to tell, but like a bulldog attempting to chase a moggie through a cat flap, unexpected things can happen. I recall a cold winter's morning in the land of South Yorkshire, and with daylight still breaking I wandered into an industrial environment that resembled a period of time long forgotten. I started my task out back amongst some small buildings, where the workers' facilities bore a resemblance of much poorer times, a sort of Yorkshire-themed Kolkata, where cold shivers replaced man's sweat. On walking around alone with my thoughts, I slipped into conversation with a man of similar age; he wore the face of a hard life lived, yet amongst the creases shone radiant eyes, those of a man who had learnt. It was one of those rare moments on life's path, a chance meeting, where we agreed from the off, a joint knowing of everything said of the past the present and with a sadness of heart the future for this planet. It continued with short statements until we arrived at a level, a knowing of the knowing, delivered by words not spoken. Conscious that our given time was ebbing away, he moved slowly towards me, and with face close up to mine, with a voice of some concern, simply stated 'We are living in strange times', it was his conclusion, and on replying with a nod of agreement, I turned and continued with my task. In short, an occultist Carnforth Station encounter, a brief moment that was meant to be, for we had shared a passage to a deeper level of seeing, and I felt humbled by the experience. I observed the other workers as suffering souls with little choice, a poor roll of the dice for once exuberant young boys who grew into men, whilst unknowingly creating their own personalities, incorporating techniques to overcome the hardships of their daily grind. Once again it could be said 'It's grim up north', and this time they were right.

Thoughts of if only I could change their lives, came to mind, alas, I sent out my blessings to all, including the pigeons who sat huddled together in the steel framework of the exposed foundry roof.

In tune with the seasons, I look to rising early or incredibly early, stepping outside, aligning, opening myself, embracing the powers of the directions, Taoist breathing complemented tai chi, then feeding the wild birds in preparation for the day ahead. 'Tis a strange thing, that the word 'pagan' conjures up all manner of viewpoints, some tainted with actions of wrong doings. Practices conducted deep in the interior of dark forests where the contents of the cauldron bubble away to verses and spells, a fearful image for a mortal. The word we seek is ignorance, and yet today I find it strange that in a time of diversity, that whenever I have visited an English school, where display tables show artefacts of world belief systems, the ones that reflect the modern age of multiculturism, strangely none display a crumb of anything of the original culture of these islands. On questioning you may be informed by a teacher, or deputy head, that there are no such things as Pagans and witches, whilst at the same time they had all become enthralled with the adventures of Harry Potter, very strange.

Raised in a land where the weather can change very quickly, and where you could go without a summer for many a year, it can and does have an effect on its people. Moods of pessimism, depression, and a fervent desire to get off one's head. In fact, people openly state with some sadness that they work all year for just two weeks in the sun. Whereas more earth-centred people, the ones who are consciously aware of the impermanence of nature. Those who choose to observe and practice the way of the Eight-Fold Wheel of the Year. Even in the depths of a gloomy wintertime, generally appear to remain content and positive, whereas others around them may struggle to cope. For to observe and practice the Eightfold Wheel brings great benefit, solar, lunar, points in the calendar every six and a half weeks. Tis a system that draws one consciously closer to the notion of perpetual change, a loving acceptance that nothing truly dies, including ourselves. With a mind for this practice, the practitioner may inherit the earth, an awareness of the changes that are constantly taking place, simply noting the number of geese arriving or how fewer swallow and swifts have made it this year. As well as uplifting, a casual stroll in the local park can be most rewarding. Taking note of which trees undress, and those that choose to stay dressed, resident birds, sniffing dogs and playful squirrels, is the moon in view today. Joining in, a process of levelling out, which in turn brings contentment, and in time the practitioner becomes awakened to the wisdom that time, space, and eternity are as one.

On entering into a new period, and being stimulated by realisations, I began to enhance my practices, and with the aid of the dowsing rods drew on a different feel for energy, they became a primary element in the esoteric toolbox.

A couple of months later whilst staying in a cottage in the Cotswolds, whilst seated at a large table referencing the local Ordnance Survey map, I noted a few interesting sites only a car journey away, but closer to home, within walking distance, a small mound with a standing stone. Without the need for encouragement, I decided to set off for an evening walk, and like a modern train journey, it took much longer than anticipated. After a decent walk and having eventually located the right spot, I climbed a gate into a fairly large field, taking note of grazing sheep way down in the far corner. A tree-lined mound could be seen towards the rear area of the fenced field, and with the entrance seemingly on the other side I made my way across. Moving closer I began to get a feeling of not being welcome and being all alone I had to adjust the controls of my senses. As I approached the earthworks from the rear, I came face to face with a large ram who stood before me. At this point I could have gone either left or right but decided to go in the opposite direction to the animal. But as I walked around, it too changed direction, until it stood directly in the path to the bank entrance. Being a few hundred metres away from the flock, the animal wasn't trying to protect them, more in a manner the site's protector, whichever way it did not want me to climb the bank. But after walking for well over an hour to get there I had no desire to turn back, and as it stood firm obstructing my access, I decided to talk to the animal who by now was looking less sheep-like. I explained to the gatekeeper that I meant no harm, and as I squeezed by it made no attempt to prevent my passing. The raised bank was a few metres in height, about 30 metres long and 10 metres wide at the base, with a much smaller ridge on the top. I sat down against the largest tree to have a drink and to get the feel for the place, after preparing myself and with rods in hand I walked across the bank top to the single standing stone. I recall attempting to communicate with the spirit of the place, the past ancestors who had once practised there, but for me it was not quite right, and I got nothing in return. Although I did receive a knowing feeling that it was my duty of call to bring about a change of energy to the site. At that stage in my development, I wasn't too sure how to break through that barrier. And after a period of contemplation, I rose and made my way back to the tree that interestingly was now giving off an energy of response.

THE DRUID IN THE GREENHOUSE

So, having lit and inserted some incense sticks in the ground, I sat down and connected with a spirit presence, and after asking a question, I was told that I needed to go away and get more experience before I came back there again. And that was it, connection closed, and with the day starting to lose its light, I gathered and slipped my belongings into my crane bag. On scrambling back down the bank, I was met by the site guardian, who whilst wearing sheep's clothing gave me a very stern headmaster-type look, before proceeding to escort me off the premises. It was dark by the time I got back to the cottage, and in summary I had gained experience, had connected, and communed with a tree spirit, who had basically told me to shove off. I saw the funny side, and so all in all it was an interesting evening's work.

My job took to me to various types of business premises, some having a greater emphasis on suffering, the main one being slaughterhouses. It was within one particular house whilst stood staring into the eyes of the condemned, I absorbed the sense of fear from the poor beasts who waited their turn. The struggling upside-down chickens, moving along a high conveyor who on becoming bunched together had their heads severed by a slow pulling process. I truly felt their suffering, as I would my own in their position, for as a human being, the ones supposedly at the top of the pile, it had a disturbing effect. But once again I was just an observer, and not a judge. Upon leaving that site with another scheduled in for the afternoon, I found a peaceful spot and took time out to contemplate, and with nothing left for the imagination, I recalled the essence of

THE DRUID IN THE GREENHOUSE

the Buddhas teaching on the truth of suffering, and of Jesus of Nazareth nailed and hung on a wooden cross. Ongoing wars and atrocities, killing for ivory, the slicing of fins from live fish, collectively as a race we have yet to transcend floor level, and it doesn't bear well for the future of this planet. We should see all animals as our own children, came to mind. But on a brighter note, being my own boss allowed me the freedom to recce, to book my stayovers at places of personal interest, and this practice gave rise to many an experience.

It was late autumn and just before dawn, the place a town in Cheshire, and true to form I arrived early for the pending job, and with time in hand and having developed more than an interest in the Green Man, I decided to have a walk around the church building to see if I could spot him. The first rays of the sun of the day were just starting to peep through patches of cloud, and as a large descending aircraft passed low overhead, the noise of bird activity heightened.

With small torch in hand, I made my way around the perimeter of the building, with the light of the beam, shapes of gargoyles could be observed. However, it was not the type of structure to give home to a Man of the Green. And so, on deciding to leave the churchyard, I took a shortcut up a grassed bank. On reaching the top I had a bit of a struggle squeezing my body past some bushes, and as my head came clear I heard a loud scream. For on rising through the torch beam I came face to face with a gentleman, whom I assumed was cutting through the yard on his way to work. I could see I had startled him, and without thinking said, 'Sorry, mate, I was just looking for a Green Man.' Well, that was it, on hearing those words, his face changed to one of horror, and with a single shriek, he sped off into the semi-darkness of the churchyard. As I stood and watched him go with some amusement, I remained aware I had just freaked him out, which was not good, and I wondered if he would repeat that journey the following day.

It was not to be the last time that I made such an impression on early morning walkers. With a strong desire to establish further knowledge I had opened myself to trees, and the energies that they gave out, and like anything in life the more we learn and practise, the better we get.

Yew trees held a particular attraction, and after a morning's drive, I arrived at St Digain's churchyard at Llangernyw in North Wales, and after a walk round, settled in to commune with the powerful spirit of the place, spending time alone amongst the ancient yew that is reputed to be between 4,000 and 5,000 years of age, I came away energised with a strong desire to develop more skills. After a lovely late-afternoon drive, I arrived at the old border town of Oswestry and having booked into a hotel opposite St Oswald's parish church, went out for a recce before the close of day. I rose early the next morning, and before breakfast made my way across the road into the lovely church ground setting. After getting a general feel for the place, and in a priestly mode with hands cupped behind my back, I set off for a stroll around the magnificent church building in widdershins direction. It could have been a set from Midsomer, for having been inspired by the whole, I made my way towards some trees, especially a particular yew that appeared to be consciously drawing me in, and without a care in the world I just went with the flow. Tucked in low beneath its branches, I found a suitable spot to sit and meditate, well communicate, and on doing so became lost within their realm of existence. After a while when awareness returned, I grabbed my bag and crawled out from beneath the greenery, and on rising stood straight up in front of two female schoolteachers, and with varying levels of shrieks, jumped out of their skins. After apologising and explaining my actions they became interested in what I was up to, they even opened up to how they felt, and why they regularly walked through the churchyard in the mornings before work. I walked with them and listened to their stories, I even got introduced to a full-of-zest-for-life man, who was also keen to pass on local knowledge, and on having filled my cup, said farewells, and with a final wave, I went back over the road for breakfast. After the experience with the teachers, although it had turned out to be a positive one, I made the decision to be more careful in my approach.

As an apprentice learning his trade, I was being taught by my inner self, open to the feel of what was right or not so, and that was my method as I followed the way. Whilst doing this sort of work, and especially on your own, you need to be brave and yet sensible, have an honest motive, with an ardent desire to seek and gain knowledge, always go with an open heart and a love for of all existences. I was now on an uncharted path, but it felt right, and it was not too long before I received a knock-on life's door, and on opening I was met by a powerful force, one that was to change my life.

It came in the form of OBOD, The Order of Bards, Ovates and Druids.

And an appropriate song.

Spirit of Albion

By

Damh the Bard.

SELF-CHERISHING AND OVERCOMING OBSTACLES

At certain times during the day, you may get aroused by that once familiar smell, a scented candle, a whiff of incense or drifting woodsmoke. Whilst in a car or walking past a shop you hear a sound from the past, one that sends you straight back into an experience, pictures of a place, people, persons from a past relationship. You may go deeper and experience an emotion, one of joy with happy memory's or maybe one that didn't end so well. Those exchanges, a negative that someone or others had said or done to you, or an action delivered by you to another. Thoughts may bring about a change of mood, one of joy, sadness, or anger, or if you are like me, generally a feeling of embarrassment. Then on your way home whilst sat at the traffic lights a person crosses the road whose appearance looks remarkably like a past friend, a long-lost fancy, then you're off again reopening the store of past experiences, memories, which once again may change your mood. In truth we never stay the same for very long, in fact less than an hour, yet we all wish we could be happy, the ads on our screens tell us so, we only need to order food by app, book a cruise, a mobile upgrade, purchase a new car and live the dream. But how can we be, and remain happy, when the nature of the universe, our planet Earth, just like own minds is constantly changing. We cannot change the universe, yet we can flow with it, and we do have the power and the means to control our minds. Remaining aware of deeper stirrings, those feelings rising from within, subtle winds carrying a sprinkling of silent words, a code that needs deciphering.

For now, in this life I had experienced and gained some knowledge of the way of the workings, yet still only in the foothills, compared to the yogis and gurus of the East. Like everything else we do in life, to achieve a goal of the highest level, above all else, one must start with determination, a connection with that inner power, the one that flows from within the soul of our being. Whenever you watch a top athlete, dancer, or musician, the one who has mastered supreme techniques, who gracefully goes beyond the range of the rest and appears to create their own time. The single-pointed desire of a Paralympian, a person of suffering, who with determination, bravery, and courage overcome impossible feats. The single yachtswoman, who sets off to sail the great oceans, she may go missing for days, physically all alone in a vast universe, battling on when all looks lost, as body, mind and soul come together in unison to survive, and achieve their goal.

For us the observer, a feeling of being miniscule, just a small child in a queue at the seaside, who with open hand grasps a cone of humbleness ice cream, albeit topped with a sprinkling of joy.

I arrived at the gates of OBOD with a full backpack, and a donkey laden with numerous belief systems, faiths, bin bags full of old dogma and all manner of homemade unseen spiritual memorabilia, even the donkeys hat came from a tomb dig in Egypt. Yet I cannot recall how it happened, I knew of no one associated, it mainly came to me in a way of destiny, accumulated karma, some may say. Throughout my spiritual journey I had continuously come up against boundaries, those demarcations erected by man to protect his belief systems and religious institutions, a bonding that became bondage. But along the way, unknowingly at first, I had collected the essence, a constant gatherer, that wild food forager in the ancient forest of time.

Upon plucking the essence I had stored it away inside a chest of knowledge, that secret place beyond the intellect, that on first opening revealed a mishmash of riddles. And like many others I had been affected by the actions of our ancestors, those inflicted upon us from an early age, and the resulting cycle of suffering that followed. But all was not lost, for the action of becoming a bard brought about momentous change, for I was now operating within a boundaryless system, guided, and encouraged to head out within, as my path of the seeker transcended into a search for the Grail.

And with a hand that held a traditional school blackboard rubber, the negative issues of life began to be wiped away. And in that motion the board became cleaner, the reflections clearer, and the stored chest of knowledge opened to reveal orderly texts. As the way ahead became brighter, stored essence weaved itself into the fabric of OBOD, the path of wisdom of the Druid Way shone before me. Having become a scholar and practitioner of Celtic lore from pre-Roman times, it was the Welsh Mabinogion that formed the bedrock, a knowledge that enhanced my ventures into the ancient places of Albion.

Protected from otherworldly forces, I was introduced to my power animal, who came in the form of a large black bear, a female that in time would introduce me to her new cubs. It may well be a strange thing for many to hear, but to feel comfortable in oneself, that inner true self, you must first learn to accept and embrace who you are, read karmic trajectory and the rest will follow. I now felt comfortable and at home with the past, for the movement of the wind brings a strong feel of connection with the ancestors of these shores, the way they lived out their lives, raised a feeling of strong bonding. Whilst being a stealth Wiccan I had practised casting spells, and like most things self-taught, I experienced the hard way by the making of mistakes. But the practice of magic and the name of Emrys lives forever shrined in Druid lore. It was with the inner grounding, the settling of roots that enabled me to venture into the physical domains of the present, and whilst carrying the key to the otherworld's, I continued on my quest. My ventures had taught me that if you require something, then you only have to ask, however, one must abide by the laws of the universe, an awareness that we are a microcosm of the macrocosm, that everything flows and vibrates, whilst paying particular attention to that of the relationship of cause and effect, the principle of joy and suffering created by our thoughts and physical actions.

For there is nothing created that did not first come as a thought.

After becoming one with the elements, and with a loving heart, I sent out a request for a staff. Once your request has gone out, do not try to meddle, as its delivery is dependent on a number of things, sometimes your request may happen instantly, at other times not so, but either way you have to remain patient. I learnt that on sending out a request you may well receive a message, the whereabouts of the pickup, but unless you remain focused, looking out for signs on the way, it may well be missed.

We were in the middle of our Cotswolds phase and had arrived for a stay in a cottage in the north of the region. As I recall it was one of those once-a-week better days, the ones that have a habit of popping up during a poor summer.

We had planned to spend it visiting a lavender farm, its tea shop, and an arboretum. It was at the latter where after wandering around for an hour or so without a care, we picked a suitable location to sit and have lunch. The chosen spot was a slightly raised grassy slope besides some beech, where a youngish yew stood almost cheekily at the rear. Having laid out the groundsheet we settled down in a Victorian style and enjoyed the delicacies of a packed lunch. A one that even included a subtle yet delightful lavender biscuit. For apart from having developed a cautious view to coincidence, and with inner work continuing to chisel away at removing pride, it was a realisation that likes and dislikes were equal obstacles in attaining a mind of peace. Whilst lying there chilling away in a peaceful setting, it was to those senses and desires that I directed my attention. After a while, the signal came that our time was up, and upon collecting our belongings and rising, my wife picked up on a gentle tug from the young English yew, so we decided to investigate.

Wandering up, behold, right there on the ground, beneath its branches lay a piece of hazel, and on inspection it was around 2 metres in length and slightly tapered, a near perfect staff. Although I had expected to find a suitable stick, this one was right off the top shelf, and on picking it up and examining, it was obvious that someone had cut it to length, but was it lost? Or had it been laid down below the yew for the purpose of drawing energy? Not wishing to simply remove another's raw staff, I was faced with a dilemma. Sitting down I spent some time in meditative mode communicating, with the added aid of a pendulum. However, I was quite prepared to walk away. But the answer I received was that it would be OK for a member of a Druid Order to take it, to craft it, and use it as intended.

One may say that I fitted the answer that suited, but it is good to have a mind that whatever aids we may use in practice (whether pen or pendulum) on having developed an attachment, if it goes missing, we may feel grieved.

However, if we develop a mind that accepts that possessions never really belong to us, and when they are gone, within the workings of the universe, it will eventually find a new owner, one who is at a stage of development where they will use and cherish it, until they too pass it on or lose it to another new owner. Within a couple of days, I also found a suitable piece for a hazel wand, and on taking them both home, and conducting the necessary work for their purpose, they served me well, and in fact I still have them both to this day.

Like a large pet tortoise asleep in a front garden, I popped out my head to feel the fresh afternoon air, for during that stay in the Cotswolds I also took to reviewing my previous studies. The acceptance of sharing those similar points of view with that of the Cherokee and Sioux Indians, for it is with their belief in the Great Spirit, the Sacred Hoop and the Standing People of the Tree realm that struck a chord of reunion. A couple of evenings later I drove and parked up some distance from the site of the Rollright Stones, my aim for the evening was to spend time using the dowsing rods, and to find a spot to sit and connect with the spirits of our ancestors. With the site made up of a number of key points, my instinctive plan was to walk a path along to the King Stone, then move into the main setting of the King's Men, followed by a visit to the Whispering Knights. The site holds a more modern take on kings and knights, but I passed that by to venture beyond that theme, a one more in line with its original purpose of Neolithic times. However, such places may hold presence of spirit from all points in a perceived timescale, and like the motion during the sifting of small particles, one is required to stay alert. It was a banking before the stones that caused my rods to react, and on investigation the place had an energy feel of happenings from long time past. After spending some time in a mode of pleasing, I felt the need to leave and push on. On arrival, the King Stone had a mild energy of a friendly chap and like the slightly merrier Whispering Knights I took strong negatives from the metal fencing. By now the circle of the King's Men had become a noisy setting, milling with people with lots to say, and so after a quick recce around I made my way back down the pathways, stopping off at the King Stone once more, before arriving back at the car, and the drive back to the cottage. You may hear it said that the answer to the present may well lay in the past, and on reflection I first came across hillforts and stone circles as a boy scout in the early 1960s. I recall a moorland hill fort where I got an immediate feel of a strong presence, but on mentioning it, no one else did, for I had assumed that everyone could, but that was a misconception.

Although the previous evening's adventure had come to a bit of an abrupt ending, it had inspired me, and with my small cog now connected to the universal wheel, releasing the brake will set the whole thing in motion, and as we know, we create that by thought and imagination. So, on a mission the following afternoon, I arrived back at the Rollright site, only this time I was alone, and whilst slipping in through the short window of opportunity I was immediately drawn to a spot within the circle. Having sat down and adjusted, on closing my eyes I instantly communed with a lady of the old ways, an archetype in a long dark cloak, one not aligned to this site. On passing a test, she gave me clues for future quests, and upon rising, and paying my respects, I left as if I had never been. Just as I was leaving the site other people of like mind arrived, and with a knowing nod, like shapes of papier mâché we silently passed by. My bardic studies had opened my mind to Welsh Celtic lore and the shamanic practice of shapeshifting, and this new knowledge aspired me to enter and explore those hidden places. And with new powers, my attempts to align my existing Eastern practices became less of a struggle, for at times they had resembled a place where two mighty seas meet, but with a course of right direction and perseverance the whirlpools calmed and the great waters became one. Yet throughout I always remained conscious of the physical pains and the mental suffering that at times we all have to endure. Which takes me back to when I was a child at the local pleasure beach, for on finishing a ride on the Grand National, a PA announcement said, 'Keep your seats if you're riding again,' before an attendant came round to collect your cash. Which raises the question, as we come to the end of this lifetime, if we were to be asked that very same question, how many of us would actually say yes, I wish to ride again?

My bardic studies took me much deeper into the understanding of land, sea, and sky. And after early morning meditation and tai chi it was the light body exercise which allowed me to weave them together in the cauldron of light. And in that healing process I developed a deeper concern for the environment, and of the wellbeing of all existences of this planet. For we are all to blame, we can sit back and hope that world leaders eventually come to some sort of agreement on this and that, point the finger of blame at industry, building construction, farming practices and deforestation, but for me the cold fact remains that there are just too many of us trying to exist in a way that is harmful to the planet, and unfortunately those in power and others less so, do not wish to give up their place of standing. During my time I have observed that people generally do not wish to know where the food that they eat comes from, those pieces of something that we eagerly put inside our mouths, for as long as it tastes nice, we do not wish to know. And as the leaping salmon lands back down upon still waters, so too the motion of the ripple effect touches the far bank, and with the fruits of the harvest of seas depleting, it is on the becoming of a veggie or vegan that our hearts and minds turn inward. A process that, if managed correctly by us the individuals, can bring about great change. Apart from shapeshifting, and a much deeper feeling for the earth, it was the smaller but no less important things that inspired me, the bardic learning of how to create poetry and the delivery of storytelling that brought about another layer of knowing, one that wiped away the myth that male Druids paid homage to the sun, and female witches the moon. As is the case in modern Druidry equality of gender aligned with that of sun and moon show no division. Within OBOD an individual may believe and follow in the path of a single deity yet seen as a religion of the ancients many practitioners follow a polytheism path with its multiple gods and goddesses, who in the main are still there to be contacted. Others may take the view that God and the universe are one of the same, but as long as we are aware of impermanence, and that the removal of ignorance by knowledge maybe likened to a snake that sheds its old skin, within that process we transcend into beings of the wise.

On my return home from the Cotswolds, I immediately set to work on staff and wand, and having completed the task, and with the practice of the dowsing rods now established, I slipped them into my physical crane bag. Along with the contents of a light lunch I set off alone to visit a local isolated circle, the one that is tucked away beneath the eastern Bleasdale Fells. On arrival the weather was bright and breezy, I parked near the local church and slipped into protective footwear before making my way up the farm track, then through a gate that provided access into a field of grazing sheep and the odd startled pheasant. The site is surrounded by trees and bushes with an outer gated metal wire perimeter fence, on having gained access, I found myself all alone in a lonesome place. A strong and somewhat strange energy moved around the site and I took time to take stock. I had first visited this site all alone, as a 12-year-old boy, and having returned a few times through the decades it had always left me with mixed views. The last time I visited was as an apprentice on the path of discovery, and on that day, I chose not to stay too long, as I basically realised that I was out of my depth, for when all alone, with a singing wind and an eerie presence, that realisation can become quite scary. By now I was more experienced, a member of a Druid Order, and a silent observer could well have seen me as the scary one. I stood outside the circle and facing east called upon the spirit of the place, and on immediate communication stated my intention for being there, I was given a rite of passage. With my trusted spirit ally in attendance, I knew with confidence that this time my deep inner fears for this strange place would be overcome. Upon the laying down of coat and crane bag, and with rods and wand tucked into my trousers, with staff in hand I moved

THE DRUID IN THE GREENHOUSE

around the circle sunwise, before entering from the east. On standing I asked the rods to take me to a spot most suitable for my work, the request was answered when the rods crossed at a point off centre, one that could clearly be defined by an eye, as the power of the site emerged. Having lit some incense sticks, and on completing a short ritual, with wand in hand I settled down facing the west, a direction of felt preference, and after a little mental preparation, allowed myself to follow my instincts of inner guidance. Upon closing my physical eyes, and on the opening of the psychic one, I slipped into a meditative mode that sent me straight down a blue hole, a tunnel with spiralling red lines and into the otherworld. And within that journey I realised that everything I had been practising, and the tests I had been given by the lady in grey at the Rollright Stones, was training for the path that lay ahead. An understanding that the spirits of the otherworld required a human to work with them, and on being accepted as ready for the task, my job was to visit the ancient north-western sites of England to physically clean up, align, energise, and reconnect them with the other sites in the grid of the flow of the ley lines of this ancient land. At this point I had already recognised that there are humans out there, albeit some out of ignorance, but others not so, who deliberately do the opposite.

Having accepted my quest, I rose up from the spot, paid my respects to the powers that be, and finished off by carrying out a litter pick of the rubbish left around the site. On arrival back at the car, whilst placing the rubbish inside a black bin liner I received an inner request to clean up the adjoining churchyard, and with some enthusiasm took to the task. Having spent some time in the windy church grounds, I found a suitable location by the outside wall of the building to finish off with a meditation session. On rising and reaching the entrance I was met by a church follower who was taken aback, but most pleased with my thoughtful actions. On the drive out of the location whilst observing large owl boxes, it gave me plenty of time to summarise the day, and to prepare for the tasks that lay ahead.

The Way of the Bard is a discipline of its own, one you could dedicate your entire life to perfecting, but it is also a foundation where the stones of the structure of the mystical castle of future learning are laid.

It was during a meditative practice that I was joined by three divine-like figures, who kindly asked my permission, to take me on a journey. And with an angelic figure on each side and one slightly back we proceeded skywards and onwards, during the long journey I became aware of other similar small groups. After what seemed a considerable time, I saw that we were heading for a gathering, and on arrival we came to a standstill in front of a wall like cloud.

Angelic beings of a higher order were in attendance. As we waited, other escorted humans arrived, by now numbering around thirty strong, we all stood with our guides facing the wall. It then changed to one that emanated celestial power, and as higher beings placed themselves around us, the sense of being became indescribable. After a period of timeless time, it was over, the wall cloud reappeared, and following a brief period of semi-mingling, with the guidance of angels, we returned back from whence we came.

The heat of the fire diminished,
Liquid transformed into vapour
the last of the contents of the cauldron turned to steam.
'Argh the vessel is empty,' said the returning young bard.
'It is not empty of space,' came a voice from the dark corner of the room. 'Then I must sit and meditate on Akasha.'
'I will come and join you,' replied the witch's cat.
And as ash and iron, cat and boy became one, the cloak of non-duality entered the room.

Des

And with the enhancement of light body and with a desire to embark on a deeper inner healing process, I took the step from Bard to Ovate.

CIRCLES IN THE SPIRIT REALM

The ovate, the one who is a seer, a keeper of keys, an opener of doors, the explorer of the inner realms, one who travels beyond the grave and returns with means to heal. Grounded by being in regular contact with a mentor in the physical realm, I required a new spirit guide to assist and guide me through the otherworldly realms, and like all journeys to unknown places one needs to prepare. With a single-pointed desire to commit myself to the task, in the standing position, I mentally prepared myself, and on stating my intentions closed my physical eyes and instantly slipped into meditative mode. Entering through a now familiar hole in a bank beneath a leaning tree, with staff in hand and crane bag laid over shoulder, I set off to meet my ovate spirit guide.

Proceeding along a narrow path, I became aware of a procession of dark-cloaked hooded figures making their way along an adjacent pathway. As the two paths met, I slowed to await my turn to join them, and whilst catching a glimpse of faces, I dropped into line. The path changed to one with high banking within a tunnel of trees, and as we approached a left-hand bend, I observed a lone figure. As the procession moved onwards, I found myself standing alone before a tall, long-haired male figure wearing a long maroon hooded cloak. He was holding a lantern in his right hand, beneath the hood a golden crown bore its markings, moving closer our eyes met. Jesus of Nazareth stood before me, and with words not spoken 'I am the light'. With a look of deep warmth and sincerity, he moved away to let me pass. I re-joined the long line of hooded figures, and as we walked onwards a spiralling circle of light appeared above the hill, sparkling rays came streaming down, it intensified as they touched and illuminated the ground, until I too became engulfed and immersed in pure light. After a time, it slowly faded, and I became aware of standing in familiar surroundings, I felt new, straight out of the box, plugged in, switched on and re-energised with the whole of creation. When I realised that the hooded figure was Jesus of Nazareth it came as a bit of a shock, for in a Druidic setting he was the last person I expected to meet. Yet the image of a man whom I once knelt before as a young altar server, the one who influenced my direction, had in fact unknown to myself had never gone away. For it was pleasing to realise that the lines of demarcation were being dissolved, but of course in truth they never actually existed. The realms of the otherworld's hold many different beings, and I now required a different power animal to take the place of black bear. The one who had guarded and guided me so well on my bardic journey. After preparation I set off, and after a little time spent in my sacred grove, I continued on a mission to find my animal ally. The path ahead was dry, the surrounding countryside was majestic with a steep bank of trees to my right, open rolling hillocks to my left, and with a large mixed forest before a vast mountain range, it provided plenty of scope for adventure. As I came to a left-hand bend enclosed with bushes I turned the corner, and there sat before me on a slightly raised grassed bank was a huge mail lion, my new power animal. And like an alternative wizardly version, the characters were now ready on set, the way much clearer, and the goal, to draw back the curtain of illusion.

Interestingly sometime later during a message session with a medium, I was informed that they could not get close, due I had a huge lion protecting me.

The seeker needs to learn and remain aware of the three poisons, ignorance, attachment, and aversion. For a lack of knowledge allows fear to rise, a strong desire for objects leads to loneliness, whilst dislike opens the doors to discrimination and anger. One of the core practices of the development of the mind is to face your deep inner fears, the ones so deep in the oceans of the mind that they are shrouded in darkness, and like giant serpents of the crevices of the seabed, they rise to the surface from time to time. For we hear the story of journeys, of how Jesus was led by a spirit into the wilderness, and for 40 days and 40 nights he ate none and was confronted by temptations of a devilish nature. So too Buddha Shakyamuni sat down beneath a tree for 49 days where he too fasted and became confronted by temptations, as Mara sent forth his beautiful daughters. So too, the Ovate practitioner must go alone on a journey of inner exploration, to venture into otherworldly realms, far distant to that of the apparent world, and yet so near.

But a wander it is not, for the lone journey into the deep dark forest is a mission to retrieve, to regain what is rightfully yours, and that is the quest.

In association with the followers of Robin Hood in the forest of Sherwood, the colour of the ovate is green, that of the natural world, the power of the green man or woman, the Green Knight of Arthurian legend. As the wise lady sat in contemplation, the un-plucked strings of her harp brought forth sounds of celestial beauty, and as the doors to the otherworldly dance hall slowly opened, the ovate slipped by on a lonesome quest.

It was during this period of experiences that I returned to a more serious mode of physical walking, now with a doggie to assist me on the upward climbs, the hills and valleys of the Lake District and the Yorkshire Dales within an hour's drive, provided openings for outward pursuits. For after spending years away from the homeland, vacations were now taken in the holiday cottages of Wales and the West Country, places that have an abundance of ancient sites.

You may have noticed that I often refer to this lifetime as though there are many. One does not have to believe in rebirth, but it does makes life feel so much easier, and it answers a lot of questions if you do. As practitioners of Druid lore, we spend time learning genetic information, that feeling of connection with the way of our ancestors, the continuum, transmission of inherited traits, and so too inherited karma.

But where did that karma begin, how far back did that first cause come into being? 'For now just follow the path,' said the waking Dormouse.

Pressing on up the spiralling mountain of spiritual attainment, the practitioner may become aware of the storehouse of accumulated karma. For the yoke of our lineage can slow us down, but by working and sifting through the amassed content, discarding the unwanted negative aspects, whilst avoiding the input of new wrong actions, unladen access to far greater heights can be gained.

Yet there's always a twist as the failed scholar resits the same assessment, so to if we do not achieve the required goal in this lifetime, then we cannot help ourselves from further rebirth, unknowingly repeating the same experiences, over and over, again.

It was around this time that I gained a strong association with the honeybee, albeit within and without, for whilst seated in the physical realm, I gained access to another. Entering through a hole in the earth bank below the leaning beech, along a spiralling blue tunnel with yellow lines, I arrived at my sacred grove. Like a garden anywhere one can choose its layout, and by now mine had expanded from a simple beauty spot, to one with a roundhouse and a part circle of standing stones, set back amongst thinking trees. Without further ado and with staff and crane bag I left through a gap at the rear of the circle and entered the dark forest beside the river. On walking along a new route, there before me a row of royal-type guards, as birch, ash and pine stood at attention. Walking on, high stone towers came into view far away on my right, I entered a place of magical flora, the forest floor was dotted with sizeable yellow foliage, a series of extraordinary large bluebells carpeted the ground, as rows of giant chrysanthemums some red and others purple stood erect all around me.

I noticed a hut, on drawing closer it had a long-pitched roof, where large bats slept, freshly chopped lengths of timber lay against the hut wall, as clear water bubbled and rose from a small well. At that point my lion guide made himself noticed, for a wolf, a dog and a horse could be seen lying down, and not for the first time an owl flew around me. A cloaked man suddenly appeared in the hut doorway, and on moving closer I introduced myself and purpose for being. I sensed his name was Alwun, and asked if he could assist me on my journey.

His face was akin to that of a woodcarving, with a defined bottom jaw and a smile that revealed deep-set eyes of an ancient. He instructed me to follow my ovate path with a subtle and truthful mind.

Suddenly with a single loud crackle, smoke rose up from a fire that I hadn't previously noticed, and from within the drifting smoke came insects that flew all around me, butterflies emerged, followed by bees; the scene suddenly changed as I became conscious of flying around with a single bee. The smoke cleared and I felt contented, then in a wisp I was back in my sacred grove.

After closing down I returned back to the physical realm, and my own sacred space once more. I had returned from the short journey empty handed, but I took the bee flight to be the key, an experience that led me into a deeper research of bees. A few days later whilst alone in my own back garden, within the sound of darkness, eyes closed, hands in mudra mode, with mind's eye open came a spiralling cane-like tunnel, a tapered basket, presented itself before me, and without hesitation I entered.

Travelling down I began to notice the odd small thing shoot past me; the cone started to get thinner, then down below a bubbling thick reddish liquid, a thought occurred that it may be a grinder, was I to be shredded and mushed to pulp? Anxiously I attempted to move backwards, and on realising I could, I felt in control. Suddenly more small objects rose from the slush and shot passed me, then I recognised them as honeybees. I went with them, flying out above a field, down into the land of the giant chrysanthemums, where I became immersed and bee-like. After a while a feeling that it was now time to depart. Turning away, I re-entered the darkness of my own back garden. When I first joined up with my bardic black bear guide, Olog, she taught me:

You fear not in the land of the living, nor in the land of the dead, or the realms in between.

The honeybee experience had raised my awareness of the present bee problem. I joined a group of bee interest and sent an email to my local MP requesting him to raise the issue of the bee problem, and a week later he emailed me back saying that he fully agreed, we have to save the bee population, and the government were in discussions with Defra (Department for Environment, Food and Rural Affairs) and things were looking favourable; he stated he would keep me informed of future developments.

Generally, the people of the nation are now more aware and are genuinely gaining a greater level of love for bees. In fact, around this region, you see numerous cars with bee emblems denoting unity of the bee with the place and the people of Manchester. Whilst it is said that one can 'ask the wild bees what the Druid knows', there are a few takes on that one.

As for myself, you may catch a glimpse of me hovering over wild meadows of blooming esoterica, and on selection entering the ones of true standing, before returning to my sacred grove with its potent essence.

Following on with the Bee Lovin', I started the springtime practice of saving bumble bees, the short-lived ones you come across struggling or lying motionless on our pavements and pathways at that time of the year. Overcome by heat, dying of dehydration, if like me you wish to try to save them, then purchase a plastic syringe, and just prior to going out, fill it up with a lite sugary water, then slip it into your pocket or bag. On the unfortunate sighting of a struggling or motionless bee crouch down beside it, and after offering words of comfort gently squirt the solution down around its head. If you discover it motionless then you may need to find a large leaf, gently scoop it up and place it down in the shade (droplets of basic water can work) before you administer. With practice each year my success rate has continued to improve, and the pleasure you get from watching them come round, then fly away is priceless. On becoming a bee whisperer, a direct opposite to that of a witch finder, it may well be a surprise as to how other bees react to you, a sort of collective bee awareness at work.

Around the halfway stage of my ovate path, things really did start to take off, having gained a greater and in-depth knowledge and practice of questing and the powers of the Arthurian legend. I became aware that I didn't have an acceptable, for me, knowledge of spirit, for when alone at ancient sites I called upon the spirit of the place, and in doing so communicated with greater powers. Yet it was the basic knowledge of spirit that I felt was missing from my toolbox. On releasing the magical boomerang, help from the universe came within a couple of days when I received a call from our gas man, informing me that the fire and back boiler were due for service. It was an annual visit and the time spent each year grew longer and longer as we delved deeper into our shared experiences and knowledge gained from esoteric practice. As is usual, we already had a connection, for he used to work with my wife's father, and had been in a long- term relationship with my mate's sister and being into healing and all things spirit that included wandering through castles after midnight, we certainly had things in common. Little S had a role in a spiritualist group that held weekly meetings in our local village centre, and the following week they were holding an open-evening event. The group was run by a lady called J who lived in a nice cottage in the square. Upon attending I was exposed to a number of things spirit related, including a request and acceptance by spirit to move a table and chair. The group were Pagan fluid, and I became inspired to learn more, and after a few weeks attending weekly evenings of mediumship, I was introduced to Reiki healing.

On joining their closed circle and with further learning and practice I became more aware of clairvoyance the psychic ability to see, of clairsentience the ability to feel and clairaudience the ability to hear words spoken. I realised I had a level of all three abilities, and with further training they became enhanced, yet I remained aware that I would never achieve the level of those mediums who had died for a short time before being revived. I was taught how to stand up in a room full of people and give readings; it was interesting to note that whenever I opened up to spirit, on being guided to a person in the audience, the messages I received were generally stronger in picture form, with whispered names and those of events, whilst clairsentience was the weaker. The practice removed ignorance, and with it, that of fear, the very one that frightens people when they hear talk of communicating with the dead. Enhanced by the questing path of the ovate, that of shamanic practice, it became a most enjoyable period that was highlighted by the closed circle meet-ups. Attending midweek esoteric sessions held at the cottage, the aim to be more creative and adventurous within the spirit realms, was something right up my street. And as the ovate continued his journey through the dark forest I was surprisingly taken on another journey skywards. It started off similar to the previous occasion, I was in a deep meditational mode of just being, when I was asked if I would go on a journey. On acceptance the angelic beings lifted me, and as we travelled through the unseen void there was a familiar feel of camaraderie. On arrival everything appeared a little more orderly, a few more escorted humans arrived, but those present were halved in number. The wall before us was different, it appeared to move, and as we settled into line, with a swirling effect it turned into water, a cascading motion, flashes of golden colours emerged, the powers of the scene heightened, all pervading as I slipped away in reverence of its unlimited power. After the indescribable, and on becoming aware once more, I was escorted back to my place of physical being, it simply felt above contemplation level. For whilst working simultaneously with my ovate practices, lone attendance at ancient sites, and with the actions of the small group, it certainly lifted the lid off the warming kettle. One memorable event happened whilst overshadowing, seated in the main chair inside the cottage, having prepared, I was instantly taken away, and found myself travelling at speed above a vast ocean. Aware of the presence of guides on both sides there was a third who appeared to be in control; although I could make out shapes, none showed themselves directly to me. It was daytime, the weather conditions were stormy and after a while travelling through clouds, I spotted a vessel below. It was an older-type ship with three unrigged masts, and as we came over the top of the vessel, I found myself being brought down onto the manned deck. The wind and height of the seas were horrendous, the crew were frantically trying to deal with the situation, when it suddenly listed to starboard and turned over, as it did so I felt myself being raised up into the air.

On looking down I noted the upturned timber vessel had a metal hull, and as I watched the ship right itself, I was taken back down onto the deck, this time I stayed long enough to notice a particular crew member, a middle-aged man dressed in dark Victorian clothing. The ship suddenly keeled over, and I found myself looking down on the hull once more. This process continued to repeat, and each time I became more familiar with the same man. All throughout this experience I continued to consciously inform the group members inside the cottage what was happening. And as the ship continued to right itself before capsizing, I was informed that my task was to assist in retrieving the now familiar gentleman, whose name was Stanley. On acceptance I immediately found myself back on the deck next to Stan, only this time it was different. The three spirit guides whom I took to be angelic became more proactive and as the ship suddenly began to list once more, I was guided to grab hold of Stan, who appeared to understand and without resistance we were all instantly transported skywards. Leaving the ship behind we continued to climb higher and higher until we entered complete darkness, it seemed like an age as I searched for light, but there was none. Continuing to remain in contact with my colleagues in the room, I had to hold my nerve, for past experience had taught me that I could pull out, but that would have implications, and as this was far more challenging than I had previously encountered, I just had to keep going. Then far away in the distance, high up at two o'clock, I noticed a small green glow, and with-it relief, strangely it was my shout, and as I turned towards the green light, it became much brighter. The scene suddenly changed, for down below I could make out buildings, and as we got closer, we were directed to a larger rectangular one, and on looking down the roof moved to reveal the setting of a banqueting hall. Inside, I could make out a group of people in Victorian clothing sat around a long dinner table laid out with serving dishes, plates, cutlery and drinking vessels, serving staff were in attendance. All appeared to be joyful, except there was no food present. And as we slowly came down the people inside the hall suddenly responded to our presence, a section of the side wall parted to reveal a large open doorway, they excitedly left their seats and began to pour out into the outside area. The five of us were down, and as I found myself standing apart with Stan, a group of about twenty Victorians ran towards us, embracing him like a long-lost son; it all became a bit frantic.

A couple of senior figures were fully aware of my presence and were seeking to show their appreciation, then an alarm bell rang within me, I was starting to become engulfed, and with an increased feeling of danger, the angels drew me away. As I rose above the scene of homecoming celebrations, the two senior Victorians looked up, and bizarrely gave thankful waves of goodbye.

We sped back into the darkness, in no time at all the angelic spirit guides returned me to the body of the person seated in the cottage chair. After a short period of calming, I reopened my physical eyes, took a drink, and discussed the journey with the other group members. My view of the event is that at some point in history the ship went down with a loss of all lives. It all happened so quickly that the people on board died before they had a chance to respond quickly enough to go to the realm of arriving spirits.

They became locked in a cycle of process, lost souls trapped in timeless eternity, continuously re-enacting the last event of their physical lives.

THE DRUID IN THE GREENHOUSE

Stanley's soul group and the spirit world required a human to assist them in reuniting Stan with his past-lifetime family and friends in the rightful realm. During the process there was a moment where I felt that I could have been detached from the angelic guides, lost in a Victorian setting, joyfully eating, and drinking imaginary fare with Stan and his brethren. Unknowingly, it was only the beginning of a career as an otherworldly conduit. For whilst working with the local spirit group we visited and spent nights inside castles, where I learnt how to send willing lost souls to the light, others were not so willing. I recall one spirit, who in his physical role inside the castle dungeon had no doubt done terrible things, for at a time of the teachings of fire and brimstone, upon his physical death he may well have been too frightened to go to the light. All attempts to assist him on the way were ignored. More interestingly two male members of the closed circle, including Little S and one I shall refer to as Big S, became interested in what I got up to at the ancient sites. On teaming up and sharing our knowledge and skills we became a very efficient threesome, for after just one run out everything dropped into place, and with assistance from the powers of the universe, our adventures became an occultist take on *Last of the Summer Wine*. To the person in the street all this will seem complete bonkers, and to be fair at times it did to us, but it is the synchronicities, the signs that you see and come to learn and understand that keep you on track. On becoming accepted a line of communication came in the form of three Sioux Indians from the spirit realm.

When in meditative pose they would usually show

themselves sitting outside a wigwam close to a fire, with the main one sometimes wearing a full headdress. At first the sightings were fleeting, but it quickly progressed to lengthy meetings, where I would sit at the fire whilst the senior one offered to share his peace pipe. And once the bonding was completed the senior one would send me a message as to which sites, they wanted me to attend. In fact, I did very little, just turned up, did the job presented to me, and left, not unlike a tradesman in the physical world. At that point I had not spoken to anyone about where I got the job information from, and it was encouraging when Little S informed me that he had started to connect with three American Indians, describing them perfectly, the very same. And in a short space of time, he began to contact me saying that the American Indians had just been in touch and they wanted us to go back somewhere we had previously been, or a description of a new site that they wished us to attend. Basically, the ancient sites of this land are connected by energy lines, a national power grid, and a number of the northern sites/sub-stations were mostly malfunctioned with some shut down entirely.

And being conduits of the spirit world, our job was to reconnect the power between the sites, which involved the studying of maps and compass, working with dowsing rods, and keeping logs, whilst working in harmony with our guides. In my experience some ancient sites also have elemental spirits in attendance, some were of a bird-like appearance and could usually be found around trees and places of water. In the main the ones I met were mostly green, blue, or even yellow and if excited can travel through the air quite fast, whilst making a screeching sound. I got the impression that they do not like to be discovered and can behave in a protective manner, but there is the odd one who can be quite playful. Our patch roughly covered an area down from the Swinside Stone Circle on the east coast of Cumbria, across to the borders of North Yorkshire and down into North Lancashire. Within the Morecambe Bay area our task was to ensure that the energy lines entering the bay from the north and western sites, emerge at the southern end and continued to the main receiver stone. One day after receiving a job from the one wearing the turkey-feathered headdress, our adventures took us to a very small stone circle in the Yorkshire Dales. Prior to that visit Big S had made a replica of an ancient bullroarer, an instrument that when spun sends out a call to our ancestors. On arrival in the area, we had two separate locations to visit, and after an hour's hike we discovered that the nearly buried first site had just one-part active stone, and after completing some re-energising work, we left to go to the small circle site about three miles away. On arrival the circle was flat, but a couple of the outer stones still had some energy, so we set up a small camp and had lunch. After which the bullroarer came out of its bag, and as Little S and I worked on the small circle of stones, Big S moved the instrument through the air; it produced a strange whirling tone, a sound with an eerie pitch that resonated through time. And whilst sat in connecting mode I saw a line of riders approaching from the north-west and they were headed in our direction; I could make out there were eight who stopped some distance away.

The front two dismounted, stood and watched. I could just about make out their dress, they wore headbands, trousers, and skins, and amazingly with Big S still swinging the bullroarer, he came over and shouted we had company, for he too saw them as I did, and after a time he slowly ceased the motion, and with the sound still reverberating around the moorland, they were gone. The bullroarer had been a success although modifications were required, but it had proved to be a most useful addition to the toolbox. Settled in, and with intentions presented to the universe, a request for guidance and assistance from the spirit world, and within the action of a sacred ritual, the small stone circle re-energised, returned to its nature. A quick scan with the rods showed that an energy line now went back to the western stones we had visited earlier, whilst energy now flowed to and from the north-east. And once we were back in the car we talked excitedly about the experience of the day, whilst recalling the last time we had ventured into North Yorkshire, for on completion of our work, a feeling of harmonious bliss prevailed all around us, a vivid rainbow appeared, and for twenty minutes stayed to the left, accompanying us on our journey home.

Our next adventure took us back to our local site below the fells. It was a lovely summer's day and as we walked its circumference, we could feel strong energy entering and leaving the site from the four cardinal directions, confirmed with the use of divining rods. It became one of those days when everything just happened, the place had a mixed feel of power with a touch of trickery and on entry into the circle we took up our places. After completing a short ceremony, I went into a trance-like state and began talking in tongues, then as the other two did their own thing, I danced through the undergrowth with the Green Man. On a following occasion whilst all alone at the very same spot, it was the presence of fairy folk, the showing of a place of entry into their world that provided most interest. For whilst doing this work you are constantly being given or shown signs, keys, pieces of the universal jigsaw that open doors to bring about alignment. My next call on the path of knowledge was one of healing; my spirit group friends were healers, and like all positive things it rubbed off. And so, I took to learning Reiki, a practice that after further training led me to achieve the master level, and like lots of others before me, I simply evolved into a spiritual healer. And with great gusto to learn, I also took to attending a local Saturday morning crystal group. It must have been an adventurous period, for with the hand brake released, I began to socialise even more when I teamed up with members of the local OBOD seed group. Upon the coming together, and with a tad of persuasion, I could be spotted at the Eightfold Wheel of the Year ceremonies, in a Manchester park setting. And the further practice of past-life regressions saw me travelling down through the pages of experience, to North America, to the ancient civilisation of Sumer, to the gun decks of an oak-built 18th-century man-of-war. Along with attending mediumship classes and events whilst working within the realms as a questing knight, I was aware that they had all started to weave into a mystical carpet of one. It was during a quest test that I found myself in Egypt, stood beside a pyramid, when I noticed a stairway. I approached and climbed the stairs that led up to an opening that was just wide enough to enable me to gain entry. As I moved along a corridor of large cut slabs of stone, all was still and peaceful which is a sure sign that all is about to change. And it did when the stones began to move and as the passage to my rear began to close, I was aware of being herded into another direction, ushered further and further into the centre of the giant structure. Suddenly the large stones began to close in around me then stopped, leaving me in a confined space and totally trapped. As fear rose from within, I gave the instruction to abandon the task, which shuddered me back into normality, and with side-effects of discomfort, sat back in the chair of my room. I remained aware of what had happened and logged what I had just done. It was sometime later whilst in dream time that I suddenly found myself back inside the passage of the pyramid once more. This time I got further, stayed longer but alas I became trapped and had to painfully pull myself back out of the quest-mare and into the physical realm of the awakened; on arrival back in a darkened room in the middle of the night, I felt lousy. For as a questing knight, I had failed the test once again, and I knew I would be allowed one last chance; I was determined not to fail a third time.

By now I had become increasingly conscious of travelling into the other realms, and during dream time whilst walking down a street in a familiar Western city, I noticed a figure of a man stood on apartment steps on the opposite side of the road, he was waving to me. Going over, I noticed he was wearing a maroon- coloured fez and on following him into the building he disappeared, and once again I found myself all alone inside a pyramid. The process of the challenge began, and as large wall slabs moved, I had to swerve around them. Having gained further distance inside the structure, I once again found myself trapped inside a shrinking corridor. But this time I was determined not to fail. In fact, I would rather face up to being squashed, and on that thought a voice from within said 'Magic' and the penny dropped. I slipped my hand inside my crane bag, and with wand in hand and words spoken stated my intention, and with a motion, the side walls began to open, revealing a beautiful garden, and I stepped out into bright sunlight.

As a questing knight inside the deep forest of inner workings, it had taken three attempts to pass the test of facing up to one of my deepest fears. I did not know it at the time, but the passing of that challenge and with skills gained through other practices allowed me to move on to a greater level of otherworldly workings.

But I had to remain aware that questing in dream time can be quite strenuous, and like life in the everyday world, we need to remain sensibly balanced.

And with a mind for sensible balance, a glance at the symbol of yin and yang, set in the direction of the East, yet ancestors residing in other directions would have been well aware of such knowledge. Toing and froing, the ebb and flow of the tide with a differential between mean high and mean low, spring and neap. And as the contents of the river flow out to sea on an ebbing tide, so too there are times in life when going with the flow may offer the path of least resistance. But at other times we may well choose to row against the flow, more difficult, strenuous, exhausting and perilously dangerous, yet it could be the most rewarding. Two extremes in a tidal cycle, yet by just moving away from the main flow, one may drop anchor and allow it to pass by. Be like water, an arrow through air, as the great wind blows bend like trees, and when the fire of the forest arrives, hide in a den of the earth like bears in wintertime. In all things, a balance we must strive, for the sound of the way of the three, resonates from grove to great forest and to the mighty oceans of our lands. And as the ovate continued his journey, a visit to the woodland of the physical world, the Forest of Dean.

With four other members of the closed circle spirit group, we set off south with intentions to spend a weekend away. The setting for the first night was the early 12th-century St Briavels Castle, nowadays a youth hostel that attracts folk from afar. It was the Eve of All Hallows, when we joined an event with a local paranormal investigation group. For the second night J the organiser had arranged for us to stay in a local inn, where the management had been experiencing some problems with a presence. As the spirit group respond to requests to solve such issues it had the potential for an interesting stay.

Apart from being a fortified castle with an excellent entrance, St Briavels oozes personality, and on arrival we were introduced to members of the paranormal investigation team who were to be in attendance throughout the night. As darkness fell, we wandered the corridors and rooms, visiting the dungeons, gathered around a Ouija board, only to receive communication from one of our own group member's deceased family spirit.

For me a memorable event came in a top-floor room, for whilst sitting down on a chair facing a mirror with the members of our group sat behind, I could see a clear image of myself and the others. But as soon as I stated my intention to communicate with persons from the past, my face disappeared, and all I could see was an empty mirror, whilst my colleagues saw me with a page boy hairstyle, and pleated white collar.

After managing to snatch a few hours' sleep, I rose and went across the road to the churchyard where I observed two yew trees standing majestically at the rear of the building. I have heard it said that angels never visit graveyards. After spending time in reflection slowly wandering around the burial grounds, I returned to discover the branches of the two yews interlinked and whilst standing below them in meditative pose, the grounding power was immense, a free gift for those who wished to take on the experience.

After a hearty breakfast back at the castle we departed to make the short journey towards the Welsh village of Trellech; our intention was to spend some time at the site of Harold's Stones, and the nearby St Anne's Well. On entry into the hillside site of three aligned stones, the rods came out, and along with the feel of flow we found the site quite energetic, especially so the fae presence, discovered in a bank above the stones. Being visitors on someone else's patch, we simply enjoyed the experience. After an hour we made our way down to the lovely setting of St Anne's Well, where a strong energy line flowed from the stones. It is a unique place with its well head and in-house seating arrangement, where two of us got the message to anoint our heads in its holy waters. After paying homage to the spirit of the place we returned to the car and made our way back to St Briavels, and we checked in for a one-night stay in a local inn. A staff member informed us that the ghostly presence was active inside the ground-floor kitchen and had actually been seen and identified as a deceased male staff member. They did not have a problem with his spirit presence but had become concerned when he began switching on the deep fat fryer in the middle of the night.

After evening dinner and a period of relaxation we waited for the pub to close its doors. It was after midnight when we sat down near the kitchen, and as a group we came together in preparation for the task ahead, aware that the ghostly visitor was that of a male worker from recent times, that the management wished him no harm. But for me, and I may be wrong, I have an ingrained feeling that they should not be there, and I for one would simply get rid of them, send them to the light. However, the owners of the pub and the other members of the spirit group held a different view, and I was happy to go with that. It was during a connecting practice that I received a memorable awakening, I was shown the front of the nearby St Briavels Castle, and in a field to the right a dark flat shape rose out of the ground, making its way across to the castle wall, and on moving up the side, entered a window. Knowing that the window was an accommodation room for the youth hostel's guests, I was informed that the dark shape was a shade, of course there are other names. Its purpose, to extract energy from the sleeping guests, and it does so on a regular basis, and I was duly informed that the higher realm wanted me to remove it. After the initial shock I accepted the task and was then guided through a process of realigning my energy to that of the level that allowed me to perform the act. I did not need to go outside into the physical world as it could be carried out as a shamanic action. With a nod of acceptance, I found myself at a spot in a field close to the castle, I was informed that a person of evil had long ago been buried in unconsecrated ground, and in order to continue its existence the dark energy form fed on the energy of living beings. And with higher realm guidance, and with words spoken we flowed as one, moving hands, actions, until it became apparent the work was complete and the shade was no more.

Upon consciously returning back to the material world, I found that my colleagues had been aware of my strange behaviour, but they were used to that. We moved to the kitchen, on entry the ghostly figure was there to be seen, once inside it moved away to the area at the rear of the bar. On this occasion Little S had brought along an electromagnetic field detector, a device that can also detect the vibration of spirit presence. On forming a circle, he laid it on the floor in the centre; it immediately started to pick up on the presence, and when we called on the spirit to come to us, it did so, and on communication it sent the device into overdrive. As a group we were far too powerful for him, and he informed us he wished to stay there in the pub and stated that he would never again switch on anything electrical, especially the deep fat fryer.

Another remarkable event of that night was a young lad, a member of the inn's family who had been fascinated by us and our practices. He was really enthusiastic, not at all scared, he had wanted to join us; he stayed for as long as we could allow him, but due to his age we had to send him away, yet I was aware that he secretly watched from safe distance. One thing that did stand out for me that night, was when I saw him much later, he had shining golden eyebrows, something I had never seen before or since.

The following year on a family holiday, we visited the inn for morning coffee. Having placed our order, I re-introduced myself to a member of staff. She informed me that the presence was still there, but the deep fat fryer had not been switched on since that night, and they were happy to let things be, job done.

Being an ovate, a shamanic practitioner, with a desire to travel beyond the grave and to visit the mystical realm of the Arthurian legend, obviously put me in good stead, for the actions taken at St Briavels were to become a major part of my future work. It started during dream time, when I was alerted by the sound of a horn, followed by the appearance of what I could only describe as a group of about 20 rough-and-ready knights on horseback. They were a bedraggled bunch, who had a Spanish-/Flemish-like feel about them, and as they gathered before me the senior one requested my assistance in cleaning up the area; the scene was so vivid that I can clearly recall it today, and with a little fear I accepted their request. On doing, the setting instantly changed, and I found myself stood slightly to the right of the entrance way to St Briavels Castle. And there before me stood a number of figures whom I could only describe as worker angels, and along the side wall of the castle the bedraggled knights appeared on foot escorting a group of about 50 captured otherworldly undesirables.

A mix of lost spirits from the dark times of the past, who now as prisoners, were being herded towards me and it seemed that everyone knew what was about to happen, except me. The senior knight approached, drew his sword, and offered it to me, and on taking it in my right hand, the scene changed once more.

A knight in shining armour appeared, and a single prisoner was led before me, at that point I thought I may be expected to cut off his head, and on immediately questioning myself as to if I was doing the right thing, I was guided to look over to my right. And there on the very spot where the dark shade had lain, below a small mound, I observed four women and a man, their heads turned; on top of the hillock stood Jesus of Nazareth, I instantly knew my task had heart. Now with a new feeling of confidence I removed my objections, and with a closer inspection the group of prisoners appeared scared yet seemed to have had enough and wished for it to end. And with the battered old sword in my hand, a lost soul standing before me, with a motion of new understanding I swiftly flashed the blade across and over his head. In doing it created an immediate action, for the figure glided towards the waiting angels, who instinctively whisked him away and up to the light that had appeared above and to the left of the castle. And he was gone from the realm of which he had roamed for hundreds of years, of our time. Then others were brought before me, helpless souls who knew their fate, some accepted, some needed persuasion, and it carried on until the prisoners were no more.

With the sound of a horn, the scene changed. The bedraggled knights mounted their horses, the leader acknowledged, then they were gone.

I awakened in a state of wonderment, it was still dark outside and I lay there in contemplation till dawn. The horn continued to sound on a number of occasions during the following weeks, mostly in dream time but sometimes when seated in meditative mode. During this period the numbers of captives had started to increase; on one occasion after hearing the horn, I arrived at the castle to find the event had increased in magnitude. Before me a line of knights in silver armour, senior angels, and a group of what I could only describe as higher beings in attendance. Although the number of bedraggled knights appeared to be the same, this time they had gathered a huge number of prisoners, herded together in a moving line of eight to ten wide that stretching way back down the side of the castle wall. Many shuffled as they awaited their fate, but others in chains whilst attempting to escape were pushed back into line by their forceful capturers. Most had human appearance, but others had reptilian form with triangular devil-like tails. In fact, the dregs of the dark world were being brought before me.

I looked across to the hillock and saw that Jesus was present, a sign that calmed and convinced me that what I had got myself involved with was for me a right action. And just prior to commencing I went into ceremony when one of the silver knights presented me with a silver sword. A small group of prisoners were pushed forward, as I swung the sword over their heads, they rose in a sidewards motion to be whisked away into the light once more. And this action continued until I could no longer carry on, the scene faded, and I slid into deep sleep.

I realised that throughout the expanding experience, and especially in dream time, I had become aware of being in various places at the same time.

In contemplation, when the horn sounded, I moved to St Briavels Castle.

And although it appeared as real as any other outdoor event, there were times when I remained aware of being asleep. Then as I became more experienced, I began to make out the natural sounds of the night, a movement within the house, that of a vehicle or a call of a bird. Yet whilst still working away at St Briavels I remained aware of awareness itself, so I asked the question, which one Am I?

And as droplets from the fountain of essence ever so slowly filled my spoon, 'You are all of those, yet none,' came the reply.

It would be nice time to listen to another from Damh the Bard. One about a Goddess who became a Saint.

Song title
Brighid.

SHADES OF GREEN LIGHTNESS

The ovate period was no doubt the most productive stage of my spiritual development, and along with a motion of healing hands, doors opened to further shamanic practice. The first step was to attain guidance, and in meditative posture, stated my intention, and like an anxious parent pulling their toddler away from danger, I was whisked away on a journey around the globe. An encounter that saw me introduced to Aboriginal Australian, African, and Native South and North American Indian shamanic practitioners, but it was to Mongolia where I met a man and his daughter. They had known all along and had been waiting my arrival. Everything felt just right, a warming shawl of what was supposed to be. Upon greetings of acceptance, I followed them to a raised setting between some trees, we entered an enclosed pathway, and after a short walk came to a solid door. On opening it revealed a steep stone staircase, at the bottom, a couple of basic rooms, one with hollowed-out stone beds, and a fireplace, from where the man and his daughter carried out their work. They informed me that it was now a place where I too could take the sick and injured beings, for otherworldly treatments.

To the casual observer the goings-on inside the two rooms would appear to be more than a tad scary. For on entry, and after diagnosis, the patient or I could be dissected, partly eaten by a strange creature, set on fire, covered with a sheet, and flattened by the rolling actions of a large stone, yet the room showed no evidence of belief systems; it was simply a place of work. As I lay down, the pair practised without ceremony or sound, and after the physically painless experience was completed, with an offering of no coinage, it was the skip back up the stairs, that brought more than light relief.

Things progressed, when one Saturday morning I found myself drawn to Lancaster Grammar School, a place not too far from home, a spot near to where the Pendle witches were hung. On the ringing of a distinct yet silent bell, the door opened, and I entered into a realm of possibility, The Three Ravens College of Therapeutic Shamanism.

It is interesting to note that throughout my life as a seeker of knowledge and that of truth, having gone through later life listening to and taking advice from inner guidance, whenever I was drawn into esoteric practice like shamanism, it felt as though a Master Chef was preparing me; one who kneads, rolls, and rubs me with spices, cuts me in slices, coats me in a secret ingredient, wraps me in cellophane then places me on a shelf in the fridge, only to take me out in the dead of the night, when new methods are tried, with further new ingredients added.

Exposure to the way of Three Ravens came in weekend attendance, and after collective circle work, and splitting into smaller groups, a considerable amount of the time was spent lying on the floor with a blanket, and by the power of the shamanic drum, entered the axis mundi. Whilst attending weekend workshops, and amongst the many, there were three experiences that stood out.

The learning and realisation of the power that the Stone People hold, particularly the revitalising effect of green tourmaline, but it was merlinite that enhanced a journey, one that brought about a meeting with Joseph of Arimathea at a well-known historic location. A process enhanced by the immensely powerful crystals energising effect on my being, with an intensity that lasted for more than 12 hours.

It was during a paired working session when one of my fellow practitioners from Manchester identified a presence, and after confirming that I had been aware of it for some time, carried out an extraction of an intrusive entity from within me. I was most grateful for his actions. The third one came on a Saturday morning during a split group session on felt sense, whilst working with an image of a lone heron standing at a water's edge in a perfect pose of patience. Whilst focusing, I was suddenly taken over by a greater power; I do recall apologetically informing the lady from Cumbria sat next to me that I was having a major realisation. For as the image of the standing heron awakened, I became immersed into a state of complete oneness, and as the collapsing wave of potentiality appeared to turn itself inside out, everything became me, and I became all things of universal godliness, just there in a chair in a state so profound that I could not begin to explain the unexplainable. I spent the rest of that day in a state of semi-blissful existence, yet one of subtle knowing, and it was to be a number of days before I returned to a level of some normality, which was a shame, as I really enjoyed it. After a realisation of such standing, I found myself much closer to the universe, one that I could only describe to you as God in everything, everything in God, myself an emanating ray, a state that some may call 'I am'.

Prior to this, I had held a single marker, for when out walking alone on local moorland fells, I came across a lone mountain ash bearing fruit, berries of deep red on silent green, the angle of the tree set against a blue sky with broken cloud, enhancing fingers of sunlight gently stroked the canvas. As witness, I scrambled through deep heather to the spot below the rowan, removed my pack, and laid down within the sound of watching crow, further down the sight of a pair of circling buzzards gentle drifted away into the cupped hands of divinity. Nowadays whenever I see a rowan bearing fruit, the vision opens my heart to a warming universe, and being enhanced by the training of the Druid Order, a feeling evolved to include other flora, especially those bearing red on green. But the heightened experience of oneness with the lone heron had raised the bar, for a breathless sense of ultimate reality had enveloped my simple existence, and for a while I remained truly humbled, but like all karmic effects it wore off, and I simply evolved into something else. And as the skipper of the trawler sits alone in the wheelhouse with rolled cigarette and fresh brew to hand, he ponders where next to shoot his nets. Should he move to a different location where the catch he seeks may bring just reward, but will his nets get snagged and torn on a seabed obstruction, or should he just stay put, and hope his luck changes? To bear fruit the experienced and successful skipper will listen to his true inner voice, ignoring his intellectual self and its ego.

Over the following period of time the horn continued to sound, in what was by now a normal setting, which was until one night, whilst in deep sleep, the haunting sound was so loud that it awakened me, and I consciously arrived back at St Briavels. Sat up with eyes still closed the scene resembled that of an action movie, even more senior figures in the form of archangels, silver-armoured knights, worker angels, scribes and officials gathered in attendance.

I looked across for comfort and guidance, relief came with the sight of Jesus of Nazareth on the nearby hillock, and below the man who always stood with the ladies in attendance, I now identified as Joseph of Arimathea.

By now the bedraggled knights contained a huge number of unruly prisoners, ushered together in a long deep line that stretched way back far beyond the castle walls. It did cross my mind as to where they were getting them all from; I was instantly informed from all points of the planet, going back through shadows of thousands of years of our time. Amongst the captured prisoners were soldiers, thieves, pirates, robbers, along with demonic beings with large ugly heads, many just appeared broken, in fact, helpless lost souls.

My task in hand appeared enormous, when the leader of the bedraggled knights approached on horseback, and upon

THE DRUID IN THE GREENHOUSE

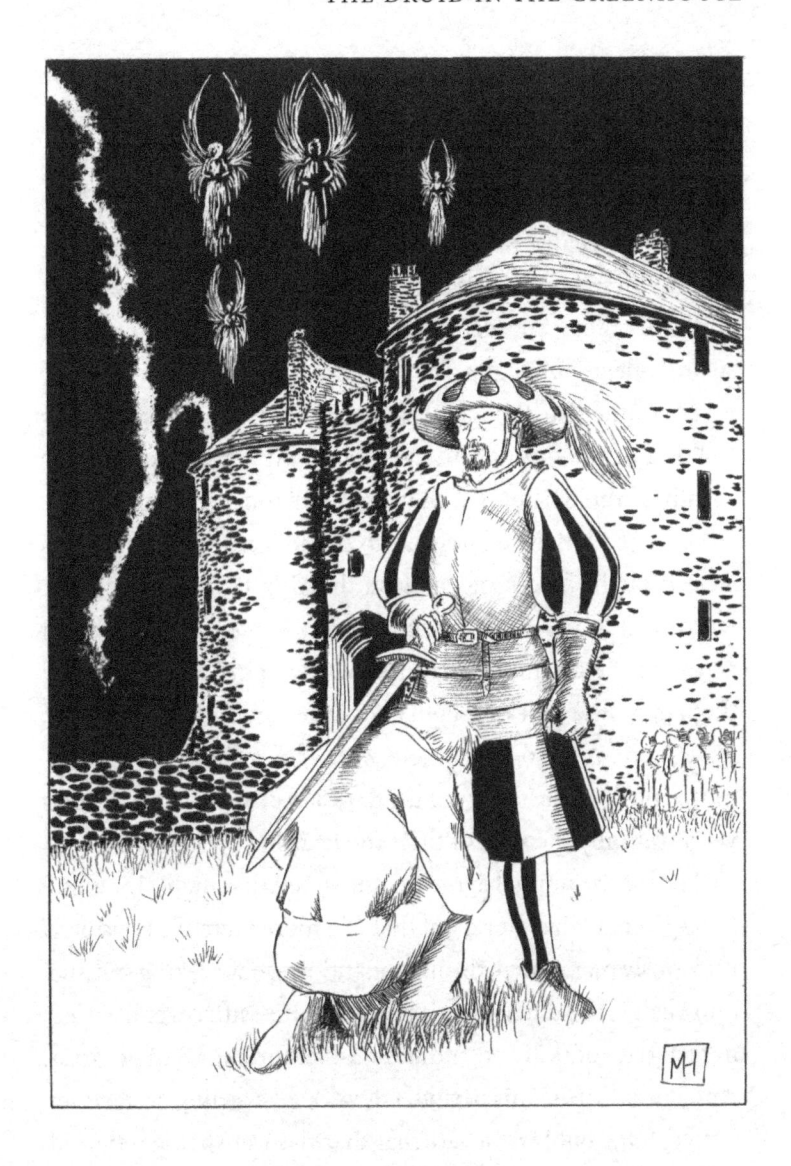

Ceremony of Knighthood

dismounting, joined up with a knight of the light, who on approaching beckoned me to kneel.

Throughout this event I remained conscious of my human senses.

Upon kneeling, we entered into a ceremony of knighthood, I found myself dressed in a silver suit of shining bright armour, and after more chosen words, I was presented with a new sword, one of pure light.

My immediate thought was where to put it, but instinctively I slid it down through the centre of my head and into the sheath of the Sushumna, the central channel. Upon rising as an ordained knight, a large group of the prisoners of darkness were brought before me, and on drawing the sword of light, with a swift action of movement the motion sent scores of them across to the awaiting worker angels, who quickly dispatched them up to the sphere of light above the right side of the castle, once more. And so, it went on, with each swing of the sword, more and more prisoners of the dark were sent to the light, and yet it was only the start of their re-cleansing process.

For me, by mutual agreement it ended that night. I was still to be given further work, but that of a more secretive nature. As previously mentioned, throughout my journey seeking spiritual knowledge, the other realms presented me with several games, in fact, tests of skill and endurance, measurements of progress. And it was during this period, I developed a feeling of freedom, not yet total, but I was aware that shackles were being removed, and like the circus juggler keeping all his plates spinning, there were still a few places left vacant at the end of the line. There were otherworldly games of testing, an occultist fair ground, the playing of snakes and ladders, an Egyptian one I believe, where after climbing higher and higher with the top just about attainable, the rung below my feet would be removed, only to send me crashing back down. The positive thing about that one was that you always restarted the climb on a higher rung. Other games came without instructions. A gyroscope would appear above me, and with intention I learnt to bring it down into my right hand, and with practice learnt to send it out as a spinning vortex. Sometimes when sat in meditative pose a large roulette wheel appeared in the ground before me, and on spinning allowed me to throw an esoteric question, and with practice this quickly developed when the expanded gyroscope positioned itself above the wheel and became a source of power.

The wheel became larger, the groupings of the numbers represented time and place, and upon the throwing of the dice of intention, on landing I could step inside and be taken away to a chosen destination. Another was the room of mixed dimensions, where changing shapes of circles, squares, rectangles hung and moved in the air. At first, I just observed, then felt that the object of the exercise was to pass through the room, but on doing, I would find myself back at the entrance once more. But the scene kept returning, I needed to interact, and with practice entered into the action of learning to shift with shapes, for with intention, and on letting go of my physical self with all its deeper attachments, slid in and became a straight line. Floating with movement inside a multi-dimensional box, gliding into a circular motion, a triangle, a swirling and evolving figure of eight, a continuous dance of unison with mystical shapes. I returned to the room of shapes on a number of occasions, until the time came for change. The scene became that of a universal night sky, and on passing through I came out into the setting of my sacred grove, albeit from an unknown direction. I never did enter that room again.

After the completion of the training, I was rewarded with a key to a storehouse of some wisdom. I took a lone trek through a huge forest of total darkness, and after becoming a bit lost within one's own imagination, the vibration of the magical bell of awakening showed me the way to a secret valley, one shrouded in a mist of green.

THE SECRET VALLEY

We are here to express our potential. "But what is my quest once I have shed my physical body?'

'To return and get it right next time,' said a voice from within. 'But for now, you must continue to cross the sea of learning.'

On receiving a universal request to visit a site an hours drive from home, I set of north with enthusiasm and a sprinkling of caution. On arrival, I slipped on my boots, and with staff in hand proceeded up the steep hill, at a bend in the road I passed through a small gate and entered into the woodland And being the only one around, the place had a welcoming feel. I made my way over to my favourite tree; it is the home of the spirit of this place, one some may call an elemental, and like all things in the forest is subject to change. For at times the tree appeared like any other, but on occasions it illuminates with an energy so powerful, it oozes pure love. I sauntered off for a while, and on returning, came across a group of female ramblers in their sixties, who had unknowingly and astonishingly for them, had encountered its powers. In fact, three of the party were so taken aback by the experience, they remained stood in complete awe. During discussion, one of them informed me that she could see things in the tree way beyond what I could. And for a good few minutes, we collectively embraced divine grace before the Tree of Love, which may seem remarkable, as the tree itself is actually dying. And as death is the beginning of life, I paid my respects to the spirit and continued up a wooded slope. It was not long before I found myself drawn by the calling of the name Ana, drifting words repeated over and over in a haunting manner, until I became seated before a small standing stone.

In communication, it was the faerie realm, the presence of Emrys, and on instinctively slipping my wand from crane bag, I was guided to draw a design in the still midday air, a motion that was followed by the sound of the unlocking of lower otherworldly doors. I had no real knowledge of what I had just done only that I had been guided by the powers of the spirit world, and my actions had been appreciated. After spending time with the powers of Ana, with a sign of respect, I rose and wandered across the site where energy flowed freely, before entering the enchanted woodland where all was well within the realm of Earth Mother.

For those of you who may be in the earlier stages of development, it is best to leave base with a basic intention, and on arrival at your chosen site, like entry into anyone's home, show respect and give greetings, and during preparation, with or without ceremony, with spoken words state your intention.

If you're asking for help or guidance, it may well not happen at once or even anytime soon, but your requests will have been heard, and patience is a rich commodity, for whilst staying alert, you may well receive telling messages, when or where the otherworldly delivery will arrive.

Not long after communicating with Ana, I made my way to a spot beside my local river, it was early evening, and my intentions were to work with the elements, and the spirits of the land, sea, and sky.

Through the ages, the actions of giving offerings by devotees, came in various forms. The sacrifice of live animals, throwing precious items into water, food and drink left at the feet of figures of deities, ribbons on trees, coins slipped into cracks of ancient stones. However, it is most rewarding to be aware of the items that the universe has left out for you, as you make your way to your chosen site. My physical crane bag held incense sticks, crystals, wand, and bits and pieces from previous workings, and on my way to the chosen spot I noticed a small shell, a feather, and a piece of washed-up string, all could be used for local and future offerings. On arrival I noted that the tidal run was entering that period before high water, so I decided to work with its powers, and that of the Salmon of Wisdom. With circle cast and whilst knelt down on the ground lighting incense, a large silver fish that I put at about 6–8 lbs leapt out of the water and came crashing down about 30 metres down river from me.

I could not say for sure whether it was a salmon or a large sea trout, but that non-subtle happening, certainly enhanced the session.

Sometimes it may be much more subtle, just a word or a name that comes to mind, an exposure on the flick of a page, a bus or van with an advert or name, a song, all noticeable clues, little reminders 'we're over here', the universe is working with you, and all is well in the cradle of existence.

REDEMPTION
At a time when all was lost, and then retaken.
Where the sacred river meanders its way through lands of no distinction.
On a bend where waters run deep, stands the tree of Calm Abiding.
As white crane stands and prepares for audience,
children born with the knowing of the Absolute begin to gather.
And as the finger of truth points towards the path of clear light,
essence of pure wisdom transcends their karmic debt.

Des

Nowadays we hear a lot spoken of the Light, a word that means many things to the path worker, for the light of love illuminates our very being, the removal of ignorance, the light of unfolding consciousness.

We are all infinite light beings who are presently existing inside human form, and in order to progress on the path of awakening, it is important that we understand that. For light body exercises should not be dismissed lightly, a practice of cultivation, which remains an integral part of our daily practice, with one that includes mediation on who we really are, those gentle workings, transforming our physical body into illuminated weightlessness.

Gaining a knowledge of the central nervous system, the

chakras, the subtle bodies, and how we are governed by our sense desires, the intellect, and the I of the ego self, as our true self remains unconscious or shrouded in partial mist if you are a morning person, then step outside as darkness gives way to the streaming light of dawn, a welcoming arrival of the new day with all its glory. Say hello, thanking the powers of the universe, upon grounding and centring with awareness and movement harvest the prana of the morning, consciously unfold, and allow your being to be filled with pure light, remain there as long as you can, absorbing unity with universal divine love.

On returning to the physical, it is the knowing that you had just nipped back home for a while, which is most pleasing.

And that raises the question, of where do we go to after our last physical breath? If we were to discuss this with a lightworker, or someone who has died for a short time before being brought back to life, interestingly they hold the same view. It is said that the state of mind we hold on leaving the body influences our arrival at the next stage, so a person who holds a strong sense of self- importance as to who they are, what they own, and what they have achieved during this lifetime, may well have created a very strong mental attachment to the earth plain. On physical death certain things may happen, we may be met and guided by an angelic being, a loved one in attendance, a person we have known who will take us to the rightful place, the rehabilitation hall for our still suffering soul. On arrival we undergo a lifetime review of our earthly experiences, our actions that caused pain and suffering to others, our good deeds that brought joy, all played out in a reel of karmic events. Some of us respond to the healing process, others may cling on to their past roles and attachments to sense objects of the earth plane.

But after a period of healing, a connection with loved ones, soul groups, a conclusion of life review in cyclic preparation for a following rebirth.

The humans are lucky for they have free spirit "yet few venture up here when it's raining,' said the young mountain goat as he stood amongst wet bracken.

'It is an urban myth, they just have a choice,' stated the elderly raven as she sheltered beneath a rock crevice.

'But why are they not taught about such things?' asked the young goat. 'But to whom would they seek advice?' replied the visiting chough.

The problem is whilst living in a cyclical existence, affected by forces that are subjected to constant change, it makes it most difficult to be and remain in control of our minds. Yet by being in tune with spiritual practice, on seeing through perceived reality, towards an unconditional level of becoming at one with universal intelligence, the shackles that bind the yoke of suffering will loosen, and eventually fall away.

Remember there is a difference between being intellectually clever and having spiritual knowing, the two appear to be poles apart, but the influence of quantum theory draws them ever closer. For some of the actions and findings being addressed by science today have been known and accepted by the gurus of the East and those closer to home for thousands of years. With a need to work towards reducing discrimination throughout the world, in my experience there is one thing that brings us all together, and that one thing is cake. However, we still have multiple variants and choices, thickness of slices, and the memory of likes and dislikes, and there lies our problem.

Tell Me

Shepherd's hook against dry-stone wall at lambing.
Youngsters' emotions, tears of frustration, unplanned actions, right and wrong-doings.
Old folk look on through stable door half-open.
Those early years, changing bedding, spring fairs at autumn as angry clouds loom over yonder hill, bowls of alms less begging.
Now I am formed, where will I go, will I be resourceful?
Friesians, swollen udders awaiting attention three-legged stools no longer in vogue.
Belts and braces thrown to the wind, one time toll gate, lies broken.
Journeys to a distant past brought forward, for like kindling the arrow in flight remains an early motion.
A time to dance, to swoon, make merry, a one-eyed glance as others wake.
That coloured mind is it mine, or simply witness to an act of not knowing.
Coracle now graceful nears far bank, slow deeper waters, secrets rise with last moult damselfly.
Hello, I took just a few short strokes to create, but countless more to dismantle.

Des

THE FINAL PHASE IS ONLY THE BEGINNING

As the green mist parted, I stood before a line of spinning discs, and with only one stick left static, I picked up the final plate, the one named consciousness.

And on creation of the spinning motion, I entered into the grove of the Druid. A realisation that on becoming a Druid practitioner, at one with universal access, the knowing of the soul's vibration, a clearer view, an understanding of the Way.

As the horses pulling the carriage became the five senses,
the intellectual driver, held onto the reins of the mind. Whilst our
true spirit self, the one some may call Atman, travelled inside the
curtained drawn cab unperceived.

The task of the spiritual seeker, the questing knight in search of the Grail, is to unfold the layers of subtle fabric, and in doing allow the light from within to reveal our true self, the spirit emanation of the Absolute.

But the quest remains difficult, for it is said that we have to live for innumerable lifetimes in countless forms before we eventually reach the stage of the carriage driver. Then how many more will it take for the intellectual driver to realise they have a passenger?

Having left the great dark forest behind, with a now more laid-back accepted approach to the otherworldly, I went about my daily business.

A period visiting listed places, halls, stately homes, and it was interesting to note that in certain locations, places within rooms, gave off strong energy, often negative. For we may live out our lives in places where violent acts, cruelty and death have occurred, the stains, the residue remains, and if not cleansed, and I don't mean with a mop and bucket, like any decay, it can manifest.

On occasions when preparing for a presentation, I have had to carry out a secret cleansing, a basic yet effective method requires intention and introduction, opening a window and calling in the power of nature to purify with love. The use of simple tools of incense, smudge stick, a bell or singing bowl may well suffice. On a more positive note, and in likeness with a field of happy sunflowers, whilst preparing a partitioned room for a presentation in a large Jewish residence. On drawing back the folding wall, it revealed a small altar setting, when I instantaneously responded to an energy coming from the right side of the room. On further investigation, a power of majestic proportions emanated from a box placed on a tabletop.

Not wishing to touch I slowly passed my hands over, and on doing received pictures and a wonderful blessing of what I could only describe as ancient holiness. As I turned the chairs away from the altar setting, people entered and the scene moved on. After the presentation I spent a few moments experiencing the power that came from the box. And within? A book, scroll of parchment, I believe. After further thought during the drive home, the experience inspired me to delve a bit deeper into the ways of Jewish traditions in Western alchemy, Kabbalah, Hermetic philosophy.

It is usual for me to observe and allow things to settle, and being a latecomer to the Harry Potter movies, like many others I enjoyed the early years and the middle stage of learning. In the latter part that some called darker, there were a number of things that struck a chord, especially those that I had experienced myself, prior to watching. For as I journeyed with my guides through the underworld, I saw creatures on the way, some appeared and felt kind, showing no signs of harmful intentions. Yet there was one particular large snake that I first observed in the tunnel leading to the Mongolian healing rooms. I began to notice it more in other settings, it mixed freely with other beings, yet it did not feel right, so I remained cautious. On enquiry I was duly informed that an ally will never show you its teeth, and that remained so, until once again inside a passageway, the large snake approached in the opposite direction. As we became almost side by side, with a venomous look it opened its mouth, revealing a set of large fangs, before moving on.

Sometime later during conscious meditation, intentionally journeying down into the darkness below the inner line of light, a practice I am well aware is not considered to be a task

THE DRUID IN THE GREENHOUSE

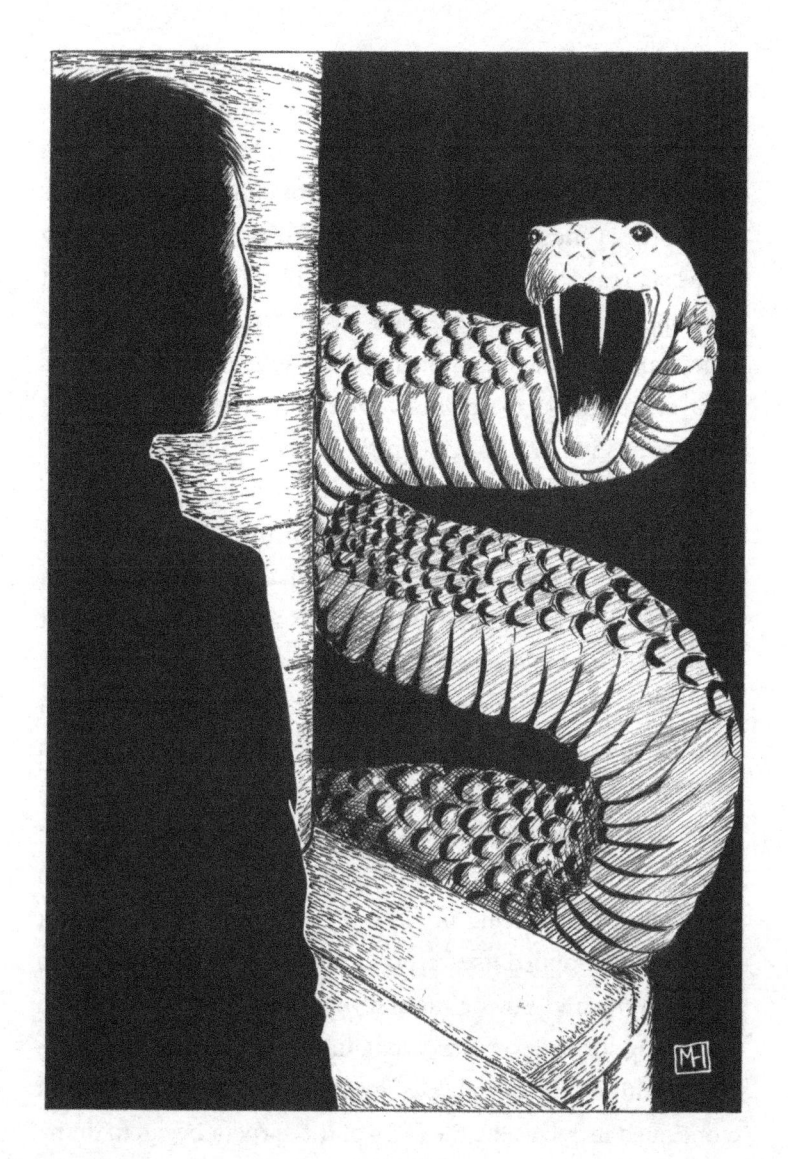

Unfriendly Visitor

of normality, I came to a ledge inside a large cavern. I had been there before, a sort of below the castle location, the setting was part illuminated with wall-mounted torches. To my right a small opening to an unexplored corridor and a couple of yards before me, a sheer drop into total darkness, whilst a spiralling stone staircase against the left-side wall led the way down. But as I approached, I was stopped in my tracks by the sudden appearance of an exceptionally large serpent, an enormous head with a long-tapered body the colour of yellow with dark green rings making its way up the stairs, it appeared to have me in its sights.

My first instinct was to draw the sword of light from its Sushumna scabbard, but I was immediately overcome with a strong feeling to stand my ground, and as I did so the serpent advanced. Its huge head cleared the top of the steps then suddenly rose up, opening its huge mouth. I instantly went into fear mode, but as instructed, I stood firm. It was only a short distance away, when suddenly and thankfully, a swirling sack containing something powerful was released from the opening on the right. As it moved through the air with magical power, passing my face by the length of a dagger, it struck and wrapped itself around the serpent's neck, and with a tightening and sawing motion the battle commenced. With terrifying shrieks, the now struggling serpent fell down, and as the writhing sack completely covered the snakes large head, it continued its job as the life force of the serpent began to drain. The shrieks lessened, as it slowly slithered its way back down the stone staircase, and with a final echoing shrill of defiance, slipped away into the darkness of the abyss. It all happened so quickly, and as a version of underworldly normality returned, I stood for a time in reflection; I felt the connection with the giant serpent with that of the large snake I had seen on my journeys. One of my guides had stepped in to assist by releasing the sack that contained something so deadly that they did not want me to witness. And so, in conclusion, the experience was a continuum of the first ones I had consciously encountered in the Sahara Desert, some 35 years before. I asked the question, was the giant serpent now lying at the bottom of my dark cavern with a severed head? And the answer came back as yes. Then could the serpent somehow return? Well, that would depend upon me and my future actions, and so the practice of Chitta Shuddhi came to the forefront.

With guidance, came a reawakening to the knowledge of the Upanishads, an essence of fruit from ancient journeys, the katha, a mystical adventure, an inward path where a young seeker came face to face with death itself, a way not far removed from that of the ovate practitioner.

Shreya and Preya, the choices we make, right or wrong actions that determine our destiny, and remember you're holding the reins, know where your heading, stay single pointed, until it is time to ease off, and reflect.

Body and mind are not separate, in fact nothing is, and if we can pull back on the urge, and manage our desires, we grow stronger, and when all our desires become right desires, the planet will flourish.

On a morning in late spring, whilst seated in meditative

mode, working through the chakras, at oneness with the universe, angelic beings appeared, faces not shown, but I was allowed to catch a glimpse of bright clothing, a request to take me on a journey, one more regal than previous occasions. Lifted skyward, a subtle feeling of joyful bonding once more enveloped my being. On arrival everything appeared more defined than before; I was met by a being of an immense power, one that some may call Seraphine. Amongst a group of the angelic I noticed the presence of three other souls akin to myself, and as we formed a line and linked together pure love emanated from the higher beings.

There followed an indescribable sound of pure excellence, and within the lighting of a candle, I stood before a multicoloured wall, an emission of pure light, those of the rainbow and colours beyond my imagination. The wall of multicolours grew in definition, the majestic sound of an angelic orchestra engulfed my existence, I was carried away in a state of I know not, and yet everything is I. As energy changed, the light sound slowly began to fade into one of a background setting; the higher ones turned to offer a form of joyous congratulations, a sharing in a comfort beyond explanation. As the scene began to fade, I was returned back to base once more. It was the third time I had been taken to the wall of the higher realm, a place I can only describe as oneness with supreme universal consciousness, and within the wall, the divine realm of the Absolute. The whole experience was very vivid. Not long after I was interested to hear Paul McCartney state how he had been taken up to meet God.

Whilst writing, the experience recalled a memory of a Pink Floyd track entitled 'The Great Gig in the Sky', a song written by the late Richard Wright about not being frightened of dying.

The word 'death' echoes the end for many people, but apart from the build-up, we really have no reason to fear our personal physical death, but unfortunately true regret comes with the heartache of our loved ones, those we leave behind. But after countless reincarnations, and even with a Druidic love for a planet with all its wonderful workings, in reality I understand that I am attached to an illusion and remain sceptical about returning.

One of the problems we encounter when living our daily lives on the earth plane is that, apart from the influence of the cycle of the sun the moon and that of the universe around us, our moods are also constantly changed by inner factors. For practitioners there are times in the day, whole days or even longer, where one can see and feel lovingness inherent in everything, even including that of a concrete structure. Then as we stroll at peace upon the sandy shore, we may observe that the ebbing tide has left behind a high line of flotsam, rubbish, and our mind responds to its visual contents. For the sight of discarded netting, mermaids' purses, dead star fish, plastic this and plastic that, a toilet brush head and even a Minnie Mouse face mask rekindles the fire of likes and dislikes, and the mind of duality is awakened once more. The formation of duality brings about unrest, the concrete structure once again appears appalling, totally separated from the eyes of love.

And it is only by closing the gap between the positive and

negative, yin and yang, that we can eventually create no-mind, akarma, a change that allows the concrete wall to reappear as one with the beautiful red robin who chooses to stand upon it, yet even that statement holds an edge of duality.

To follow the path of right view, thought, speech and action is also the Druid Way, for the hugging of a tree involves effort, a sharing, touched by the individual rays of the same sun, the mirror of the moon, for bonding with another life form, brings forth contentment and wellbeing.

For in that process, the worlds are drawn together, the sheaths of the realms fall back and reveal their truths, and as we step out from its within, we enter a new world, refreshed, and awakened, another foothold on the next rung up the ladder of spiritual attainment or put another way a climb through the chakras.

Springtime arrives with a canvas of true colours, drawing us away from the recess of winter, a positive calling to awakening souls.

The setting of goals, going away, sleeping on the ground to be embraced by Earth Mother, sitting on a rock beside a fall of water, bare feet submerged in mountain pool. Climbing high with expanding horizons, touched by droplets of subtle rain carried on warm breeze, the presence of the eternal, as mortals perceive the infinite. 'But what is the difference between a thought and a feeling?' asked the young seeker. Well, basically its mind before matter, yet the imbalance of head and body plays a major role in our daily lives, for we often hear the phrase 'my head is telling me not to go there, but my heart says please we must'. But they cannot both be right. So, who should I believe, who can I turn too? We could consult the oracle but we may live a long way from Mongolia; a true medium may assist or we could use a spiritual aid like a crystal pendulum, putting the question to our true selves. For upon questioning, the young seeker unfolds spiritual knowledge, and from knowledge, knowing and from the universal mind comes the known of wisdom. 'Tap into the Akashic records,' a wise Russian Madame once proclaimed. For it is with the integrated view of heart and mind, and that of Atman, the spiritual essence of the divine within, that our questions can be truly answered. And at that point of progression, we may well shed the shackles of attachment, lay down the pendulum, the cards, put aside those physical aids and proceed on the journey with a universal wholeness.

During the years prior to Covid-19 restrictions, we formed a small seed group named The Corvids, a gathering of myself and two witches, J & M from the same coven who are both members of OBOD.

At meets we drew on our holding of vision, hearing, sensing and clear knowing. The experience of brain waves, theta, alpha, beta and gamma, Sanskrit teachings of maya, imagination, intuition, awareness, relative and absolute truth and on emptiness, the lack of inherent existence.

How come the figure on the Gundestrup Cauldron appears to be that of Shiva? During this period my completion of the final grade came about, and with a need to fill the void, and give something back, I pledged to write this book. Meanwhile at meets our attention turned to the physical and the subtle, the awakening call of the cosmic vibration of Awen, a journey through the chakras, astral body with its sheaths of prana, mind, intellect with mantra meditations from root to the mind's eye, the seed body, and joyful bliss.

Apart from regular seed group meets I spent a very enjoyable and informative 12 months learning astrology, taught by a knowledgeable wise lady at her local home. Apart from open Saturday events, the true benefits came from weekly group attendance with like-minded folk.

The effort put in was knowledge gained, but the gift of essence came from a deeper learning of myself. For it was interesting to discover that although we are born with three attributes, that of planetary alignment, accumulated karma, and free choice it those subtle traits, that with conscious practice of inner development and awareness, the bondage of assumed fixed traits of personality can soften and, in some cases, can almost go away. It is also interesting to note that you may well have inherited similar behaviour patterns to those of old Uncle Archie or great-great-Grandma Evelyn. 'But how can that be? For I never met them,' asked the young lady preparing the soup.

'It is evolutionary memory, accumulated genetic karma at play,' said the chef from the East.

One night during the midweek attendance, whilst taking a tea and cake break, the group got into a discussion on where we are heading in terms of spiritual awakening as a whole. As usual it was based on a positive approach, and as everyone opened up, I became awakened with a vision, one I described to the room, pictures, soft words of world disasters, that of fire, of major floods, a sweeping world plague and a serious war. I was aware that I had just brought the room down, including myself, but alas, unfortunately it came into being.

But nothing can happen without an action, a celestial happening, a Saturn–Pluto conjunction.

After catching Covid-19 early on, I went on to develop whooping cough, *Bordetella pertussis*, a disease I suffered from as a small boy. But after months of feeling weak and lethargic, in a strange way, I actually enjoyed the Covid experience. A period of plane-less skies and traffic-less roads, observing nature take a break from its constant hammering, was a pleasurable experience.

Sadly, people died and many struggled, but a lot slowed down to take on a more leisurely pace. Working from home, a time to reflect, changes in lifestyle, perhaps a move away, being nicer to others, putting family first. For some it simply wore off, but for others not so, and if you switch off from politics and the intensity of the agenda-based media, the pace has slowed, values are changing, a bowl of what was once is now not so, is there to be sampled. And as life moves on, I find myself in a new local OBOD seed group, attending regular Tai Chi - Qi Gong classes, and fortnightly gatherings with a local group of soul friends.

A Call at Dawn

As I kneel before the Cauldron of Wisdom.
Felt sense, as contents evaporate and merge with air,
forever rising, layers of subtle matter disperse to aether.
Absorbed in mind by mantra sung, red becomes violet,
the hooded serpent envelops my being.

Des

THE KNOWING OF THE KNOWN

I have a long-time friend, like me a seeker, and as the two trains travelled at the same speed in opposite directions, the route to my destination crossed the spiritual heartlands, whilst his took a scenic yet more scientific route.

There were times when the two trains pulled into a junction station, notes and experiences shared, although of interest, brought little attainment.

Then after decades of travelling through a different space and time zone came a game changer, the learning of how a beam of electrons is affected when watched by a quantum observer, and the two edged closer.

As every cell has its own intelligence, we travel towards a single track. Will they come together as one, or crash and create a new universe?

We can extend the range of observation, endeavour to discover the theory of everything with a single equation, a formula that fills the hole.

Subjective and objective two horns on the same goat.

'But how can something emerge from nothing, and then

order arrive from chaos?' asked the Mad Hatter, as he helped himself to another slice of quark.

"'Tis a matter of the observer effect,' said the alert Dormouse.

The brain, my father called grey matter when he wanted me to use it, not to be confused with the mind, but the matter that mind substance manifests itself.

After many years of observing mind, being conscious that my true self does not remain buried in the ground or burnt on physical death.

I concluded that my own mind was a part of the same something on a much grander scale, for in yogic philosophy individual minds are shielded from universal mind by thin layers of matter. In Dharmic traditions a closed lotus flower provides an example. Within continuous conscious meditation practice the petals of the flower slowly unfold, as the layers of matter fall back it provides an increased level of communication with universal mind, one that is yet to be formulated into mathematics. For upon the action of unfoldment or opening of the petals of the lotus, it reveals the higher or true spirit self, illumination, a halo present, nirvana within and without.

But until I achieve that quest, I will remain seated in samsara.

But, hey, chin up, we're here, let us embrace the beauty of the planet, a joyful sampling of her treasures.

And as the boy wizard closed the greenhouse door for the final time, he unknowingly stepped out onto the way of the great universe.

Elsie's Pantry

Cast take a bow, faces wiped clean, disrobed garments on coloured hangers, fire curtain kisses stage floor.
Audience rise, proceed on foot, tram, cab or one for the road in merriment alley.
Turning of keys, hands move, fingers touch, room doth brighten.
A simple act, pots away, waste bins emptied.
For it all starts again tomorrow.

I will leave you for now with a George Harrison Indian inspired song.
from the *SGT Pepper* album:

'Within You Without You'.

Blessings to You All.

Des